Imen Ghadhab
Haifa Bergaoui
Dhekra Toumi

MALIGNANT GERM CELL TUMOURS OF THE OVARY

Imen Ghadhab
Haifa Bergaoui
Dhekra Toumi

MALIGNANT GERM CELL TUMOURS OF THE OVARY

ScienciaScripts

Imprint

Cover image: www.ingimage.com

This book is a translation from the original published under ISBN 978-620-6-71210-7.

Publisher:
Sciencia Scripts
is a trademark of
Dodo Books Indian Ocean Ltd. and OmniScriptum S.R.L publishing group

120 High Road, East Finchley, London, N2 9ED, United Kingdom
Str. Armeneasca 28/1, office 1, Chisinau MD-2012, Republic of Moldova, Europe
Printed at: see last page
ISBN: 978-620-8-08167-6

Contents

1 Introduction

germ cell tumours of the ovary are the rarest *of the* most common ovarian tumours and are estimated to account for 6% of all ovarian tumours [1]. They are malignant in only 5% of cases [1], and malignant germ cell ovarian tumours (MGOT) are exceedingly rare, representing only 2% to 3% of malignant ovarian tumours [2].

Histologically, malignant germ cell tumours of the ovary are composed of several tumour types and are divided into two groups:

- malignant seminomatous germ cell tumours: dysgerminoma.
- non-seminomatous malignant germ cell tumours (NSMGCTs) which are histologically defined by the presence of at least one of the following contingents: yolk sac tumour, choriocarcinoma, embryonal carcinoma and immature teratoma.

From a diagnostic, therapeutic and prognostic point of view, MCTs differ from adenocarcinomas in a number of ways:

✓ The age of onset is much earlier, since these tumours occur in girls and young women [3] and are the most common cancer in women before the age of 20,

✓ Diagnosis at an earlier stage,

✓ The prognosis is much better, with a 5-year survival rate of 100% for seminomatous TGMO and 85% for non-seminomatous TGMO [4],

✓ Very high chemosensitivity,

✓ Specific markers differ according to histological type,

✓ And specific treatment modalities, with surgery that is usually conservative and chemotherapy protocols that are adapted [3].

The standard treatment for GIST includes fertility-preserving surgery, defined as preservation of at least one adnexa and the uterus, followed by adjuvant chemotherapy of the BEP type (combining blemomycin, etoposide, cisplatin) except for stage IA pure dysgerminoma and grade 1 immature teratoma for which surgery alone represents the treatment of choice. [5]

However, certain issues in the management of GIST remain unresolved to date, such as the role of complete surgical staging [6] and the degree of completion of staging surgery in early stage GIST; the role of secondary reduction surgery in patients with recurrent or progressive GIST; the role of surveillance in stage IA GIST [6] and finally the role of neoadjuvant chemotherapy in the management of advanced GIST [7, 8].

In addition, very few Tunisian studies have analysed the diagnostic features of this type of tumour, as well as the therapeutic and evolutionary methods, whereas the rarity and management difficulties justify a centralised study on the management strategy for patients presenting with a malignant germ cell ovarian tumour.

To this end, we have carried out this study and set ourselves the following objectives:

■ To report and analyse the epidemiological, diagnostic, anatomopathological, therapeutic and prognostic features of malignant germ cell tumours of the ovary illustrated and treated in the Gynecology-Obstetrics Department of the Farhat Hached

University Hospital in Sousse.

- Compare our results with the literature.
- Propose a decision-making diagram to improve management of this condition in the Tunisian context.

2 Patients and methods

I. Type and population of study

1. Type of study

This is an observational, retrospective, descriptive and analytical study.

2. Study period

The study period is 21 years, from 1 September 1998 to 30 September 2019.

3. Location of the study

The study was carried out in the Gynecology-Obstetrics, Medical Carcinology and Anatomopathology departments of the FARHAT HACHED University Hospital Centre (CHU) in Sousse.

4. Study population

The study included all patients managed for histologically confirmed malignant germ cell tumours of the ovary.

II Sampling

1. Inclusion criteria

> Patients with a histologically proven malignant germ cell tumour of the ovary.

> Histological type: dysgerminoma, yolk sac tumour, choriocarcinoma, embryonal carcinoma and immature teratoma, mixed germ cell tumour.

2. Non-inclusion criteria

❖ Other histological types: cancerised mature teratoma

Files that cannot be used.

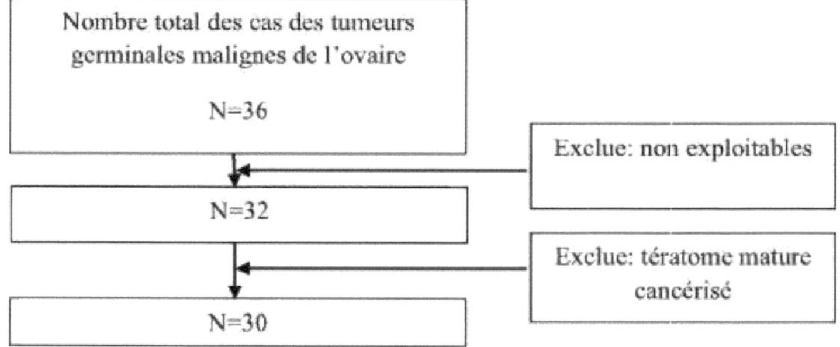

General diagram of the study (in French)

3. Size of workforce

A total of 30 files were eligible for our study.

III. Definition of study variables

The main explanatory variables studied were: (Appendix 1)

- Epidemiological data: age, parity.
- Carcinological antecedents.
- Clinical data: consultation time; circumstances of discovery; tumour size.
- Radiological data.
- gross and histological anatomopathological data.

- Therapeutic therapeutics : surgery, chemotherapy.
- data.

IV. Data collection

The data collection method was based on the use of medical records, patients' operative and anatomopathology reports and adjuvant treatment reports (chemotherapy) transcribed on a pre-established computerised form (**Appendix 1**).

V. Statistical methodology

The data collected was both quantitative and qualitative.

A descriptive statistical analysis was carried out on the main sociodemographic, clinical and therapeutic variables studied: qualitative data will be expressed as numbers and percentages, quantitative data as means and standard deviations.

All this data was entered and processed using SPSS version 24.0 software.

Survival was calculated using the Kaplan-Meir method.

VI. Data from the literature

A bibliographic search was carried out using the search engines Pubmed/Medline, Science Direct, Google Schoor, Google Books and Cochrane datasse. The search used the following keywords:

Ovary", "Malignant Germ Cell Tumors", "Management", "Conservative Surgery", "Radical Surgery", "Chemotherapy", "Staging", "Prognosis" and "Fertility".

3 Results

A. Overall results of the series

I. Epidemiological profile

1. Incidence

30 cases of malignant germ cell tumours of the ovary (MGCT) were identified during the study period.

During the same period, 717 cases of malignant ovarian tumours were recorded in our Gynecology and Obstetrics Department at CHU Farhat Hached.

In relation to the total number of malignant ovarian tumours, the incidence of TGMO was 4.1%.

2. Workforce

Over a period of 21 years, 30 cases of malignant germ cell tumours of the ovary at different stages of progression were recorded, with a variable distribution depending on the year.

3. Age

The average age was 22, with extremes ranging from 10 to 40.

The two age groups most affected were 20 to 24 and 30 to 34 (Figure 1).

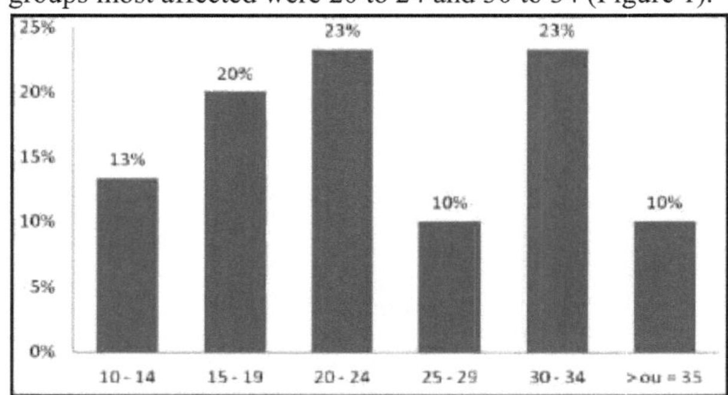

Figure 1 : Breakdown of patients by age group

The mean age varied according to histological type. In fact :

- For dysgerminomas, the mean age was 17 years (10 to 31 years).

Table I: Age according to histological type.

Histological type	Medium	Minimum	Maximum
Dysgerminoma	17	10	31
TGMND	25	13	40

- The mean age of non-dygerminomatous tumours was 25 years, with extremes ranging from 13 to 40 years (Table I-II).

Table II: Age by TGMND histological subtypes

Histological type	Average (years)	Minimum	Maximum

Embryonal carcinoma	**23**	**13**	**31**
Immature teratoma	**25**	**14**	**40**
Yolk sac tumour	**35**	**35**	**35**
Mixed germ cell tumours	**16**	**16**	**16**

4. Antecedents

4.1. Family history

In our series, no patients had a family history of ovarian cancer, and only one patient had a family history of non-Hodgkin's lymphoma in a paternal uncle.

4.2. Personal history

In our study, none of the patients had been treated for gynaecological or other cancers.
Surgical antecedents were found in 6 cases; a right cystectomy for a mature teratoma of the ovary was performed in one patient, a cesarean delivery in 2 patients, a tonsillectomy in one and an appendectomy in 2 patients.
Hypertension and diabetes were the only medical antecedents found in our study. (Figure 2).

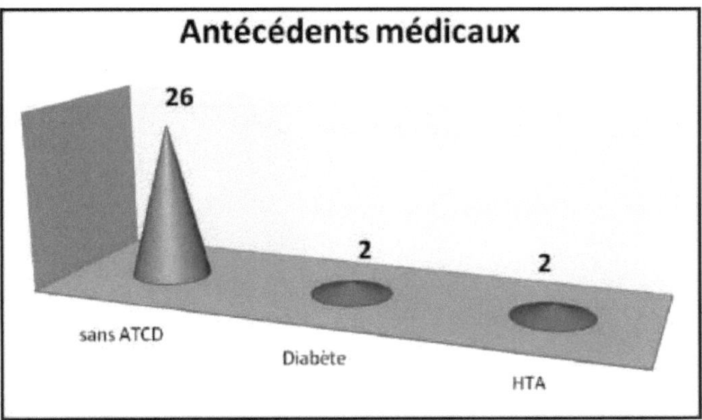

Figure 2: Breakdown of patients by medical history

4.3. Gyneco-obstetrical status

Two of our patients, aged 10 and 12, were in their first pregnancy.
The majority of patients were genitally active (28 cases), and none were menopausal.
The average age at menarche was 12.9, with extremes ranging from 11 to 15.
Of the patients with active genitalia, 8 were married (27%), one of whom was being treated for 2 years of primary infertility.
Most of our candidates (22 patients, 73%) were single.
(Figure 3)

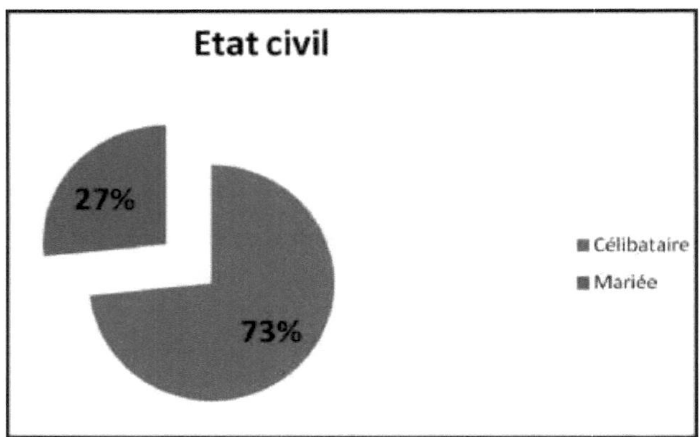

Figure 3: Distribution of patients by marital status

The averages for gestation and parity in these patients were 1.6 (0 to 7) and 1.2 (0 to 4) respectively.

In our series, 6 patients (20%) were using non-hormonal contraception and 2 patients (7%) were using hormonal contraception. (Figure 4)

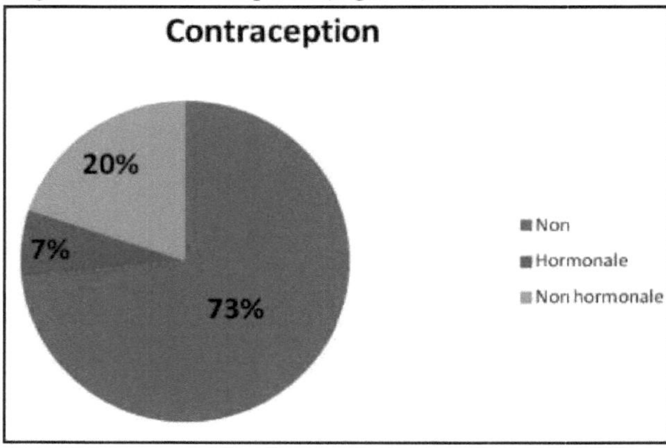

Figure 4: Breakdown of patients by contraceptive method

II. Clinical Study

1. Circumstances of discovery

1.1. Warning signs

Abdominopelvic pain was the main complaint in 45% of cases (24 patients).

Acute abdominal symptoms were observed in one patient and the etiology was adnexal torsion.

The 3 other main clinical signs that brought patients to the clinic were an increase in abdominal volume in 17% of cases, a change in general condition in 11% of cases and palpation of an abdominal mass in 11% of cases.

In one patient, it was discovered by chance during the investigation of a deep vein

thrombosis.
The least frequently observed signs were transit and urinary disorders.

One patient presented with a menometrorrhagia-like cycle disorder.
(Figure 5).
The combination of increased abdominal volume and abdominopelvic pain dominated the clinical picture.

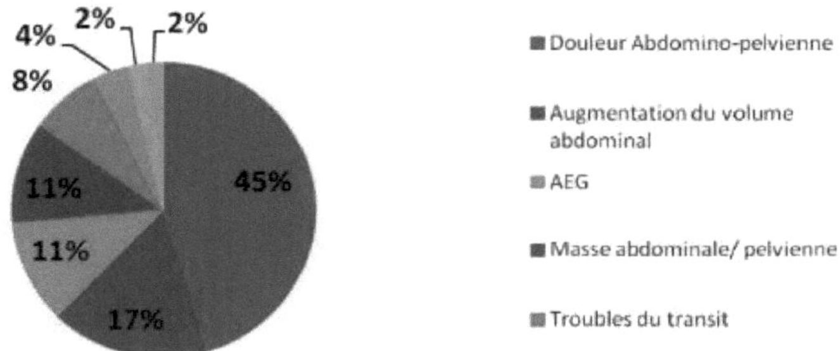

Figure 5: Breakdown of patients by reason for consultation

1.2. The consultation deadline

In our series, the average time between the appearance of the first signs and the date of consultation was 3 months, with extremes ranging from 15 days to 12 months.
Delays in consultation before 6 months represented 87% of cases and 13% of cases after 1 year (Figure 6).

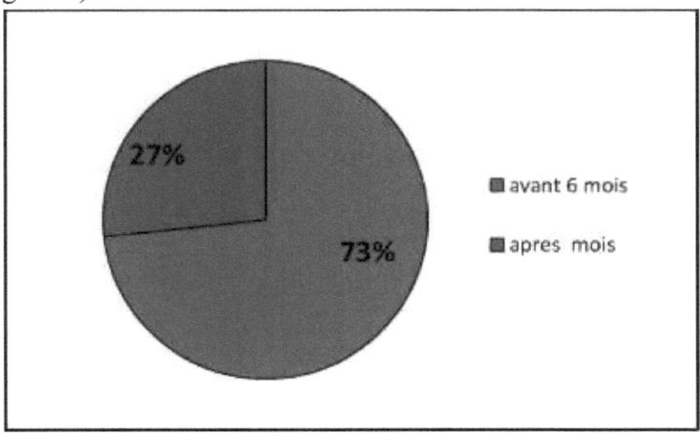

Figure 6: Breakdown of patients by length of consultation

III. Explorations

1. Tumour markers

- The alpha-lci'to-proteine (AFP) assay was performed in 22 patients: it was pathological in 15 (68%). These were immature teratoma in 6 patients, dysgerminoma in 3 patients, vitelline tumour in 3 patients, embryonal carcinoma in 2 and mixed TG in the last (Figure 7 and 8).

The highest levels were observed in yolk tumours (with a maximum level of 61278 ng/ml and a minimum of 1615 ng/ml).

- Chorionic Gonadotropic Hormone (CGH) was measured in 6 patients: 2 were pathological, one a dysgerminoma and the second a vitelline tumour.
- Similarly, Lactate DesHydrogenase (LDH) was measured in 4 patients and was pathological in 1.
- However, the CA125 assay was performed in the majority of cases (70%), and was pathological in 100% of cases. (Figure 7).

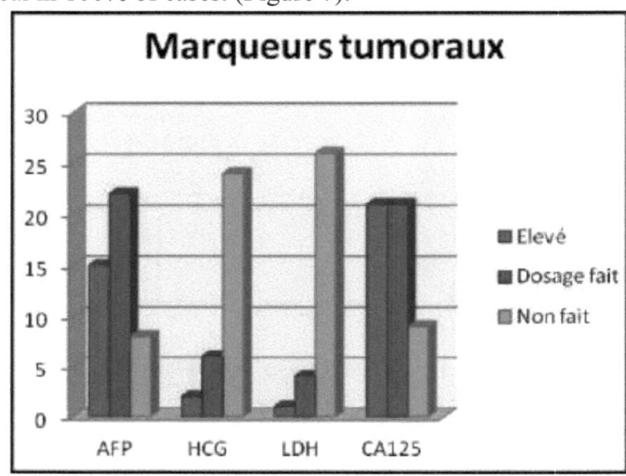

Figure 7: Tumour marker assay

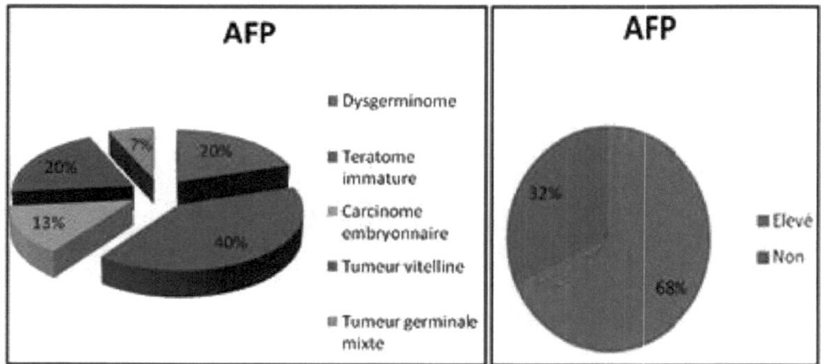

- **Figure 8: AFP positivity and distribution according to histological type**

2. Radiological investigations

2.1. Abdominopelvic ultrasound

Preoperative ultrasound was performed in 24 patients (80%). It showed a right pelvic mass in 50% of cases, a left pelvic mass in 33% of cases and a bilateral pelvic mass in 13% of cases. (Figure 9)

In 2 cases, the location of the tumour could not be determined due to the size of the tumour.

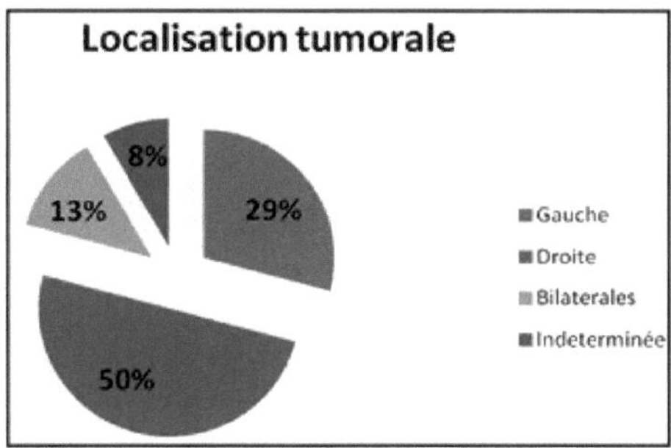

Figure 9: Tumour laterality

Ultrasound showed a solid cystic image in 16 cases (66.7%). The mass was heterogeneous in appearance in 21 cases, thickened with its own wall in 13 cases and often echogenic (9 cases).

In more than half the cases, these masses were hyper-vascularised with intense Doppler imaging (Figure 10).

The mean tumour size at diagnosis was 140 mm, with extremes of 60 and 280 mm.

With regard to ultrasound signs of malignancy, septations were rarely objective in our series (5 cases) and endocystic vegetations much less so (one case).

Ultrasound also showed ascites in 9 cases and peritoneal nodules suspected of malignancy in 2 cases.

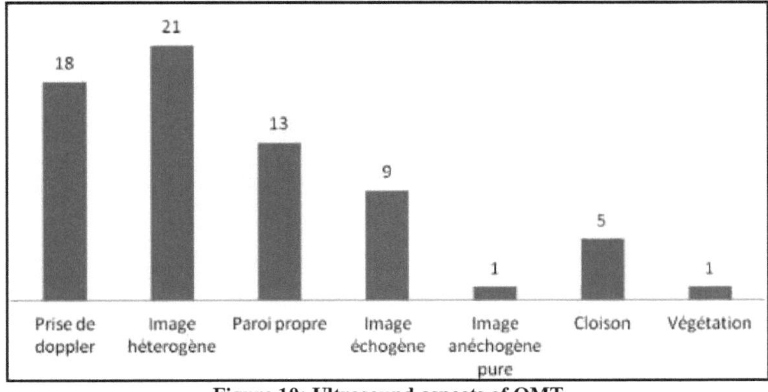

Figure 10: Ultrasound aspects of OMT

2.2. Thoracic-abdominal-pelvic computed tomography (CT)

This examination was only carried out in 11 patients, in 2 of whom there was doubt as to the exact origin of the tumour, and in the other cases the tumour was larger than 150 mm.

CT confirmed the ultrasound findings, showing heterogeneous tumours in 10 cases, 7 of which were immature teratomas, and tissue and fat in 5 cases. Right urethral dilatation was seen in 2 cases.

As part of the extension work-up, CAT scans did not show any peritoneal, hepatic or pulmonary tumours of secondary origin, or lymph node involvement in all cases.

2.3. Magnetic resonance imaging (MRI)

MRI was only performed in five patients: 2 cases of immature teratomas, one case of dysgerminoma, one case of vitelline tumour and one case of embryonal carcinoma.

In the 2 cases of immature teratomas, the tumour formation was a heterogeneous T2 hyper signal containing partitions.

In the case of dysgerminoma, the mass was heterogeneous, containing areas of T1 hyposignal and T2 hyper signal.

Other signs of malignancy were absent, apart from an effusion in 2 cases, which was free and of small size.

IV. surgical treatment

In our study, all our patients initially underwent a surgical procedure with a dual diagnostic and therapeutic aim.

Given the volume of the tumour, 21 patients were approached by midline laparotomy, and 9 by crelioscopy, 3 of which were converted to laparotomy. (Figure 11)

The average time between the initial operation and the date of the first consultation was 19 days, with extremes ranging from 01 day to 60 days.

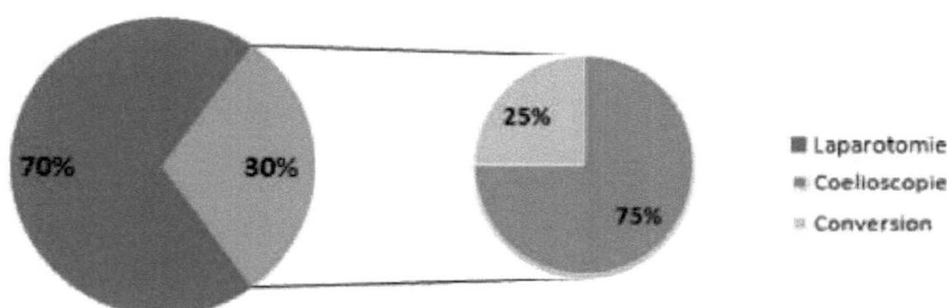

Figure 11: Surgical approaches

1. Operational findings

The tumour mass ëtended to be solid-cystic in 60% of cases, solid in 30% and cystic in 10%. (Figure 12)

The tumour formations had a clean wall in 26.6% of cases.

Exocystic vëgëtations ëwere present in 13.3% of cases and septations in 10% of cases. (Figure 12)

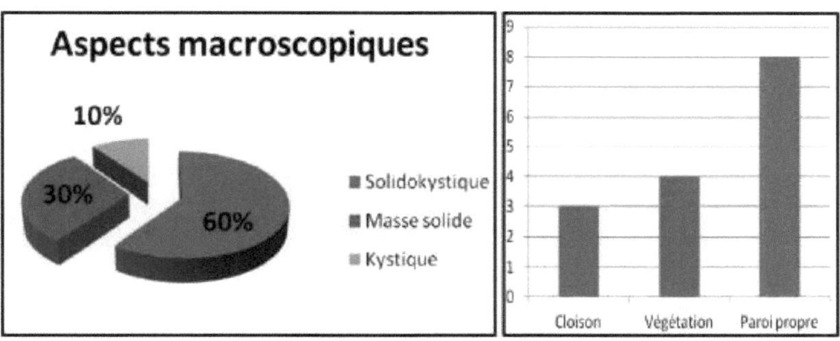

Figure 12: Macroscopic aspects of surgical findings

Ascites ë!^^ present in 24 patients (80%); it ë!^^ free and not partitioned in all cases. The effusion was small in 73% of cases,
medium abundance in 17% of cases and high abundance in 8%. (Figure 13).

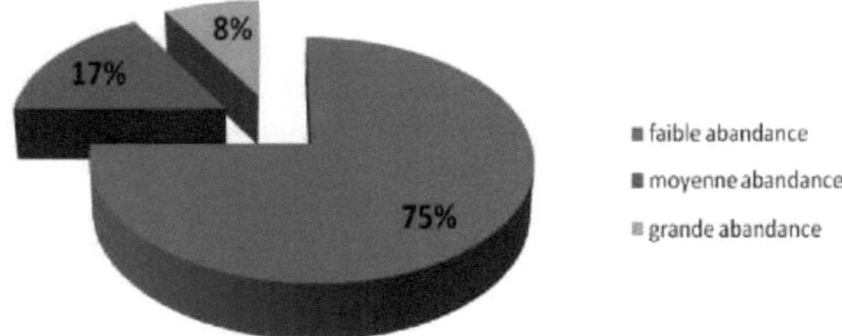

Figure 13: Assessment of effusion

Peritoneal nodules were found in 10 patients in the following locations: cul de sac of Douglas, parietal peritoneum, visceral perivesical, on the epiploon and in the parietocolonic gutters.

Intraoperatively, the tumours were classified as stage Ia in 33% of cases, Ib in 7%, Ic in 20%, IIIb in 13% and IIIc in 27%. (Figure 14)

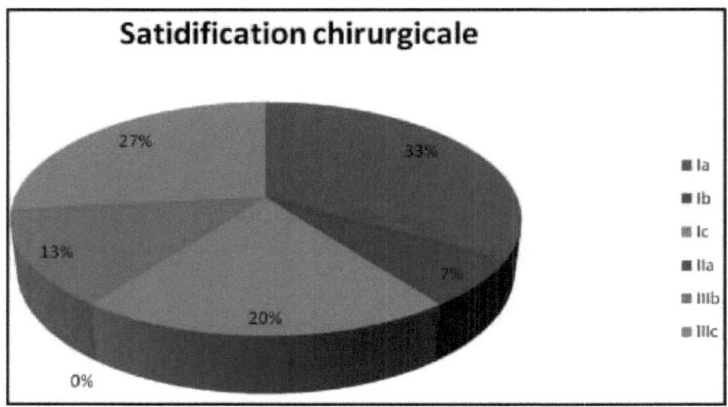

Figure 14: Distribution of patients according to surgical staging

2. Operating procedures

Peritoneal cytology was the first procedure performed in 28 patients (93.3%).

For stage I, the initial surgical treatment was conservative, leaving an ovary and uterus in place in 16 patients (94.1%), and radical embolism in one patient (5.9%). (Table III)

For stage II, 100% of patients underwent conservative treatment.

Contralateral ovarian biopsy and peritoneal biopsies were not performed in all stage I and II cases.

The procedures performed for stage III tumours were ovarian biopsy in 63.3% of cases, adnexectomy in 36.3% and peritoneal biopsies in 90.9% of cases.

Ovarian biopsy was bilateral in 71.4% of cases. (Figure 15).

Table III: Surgical procedures performed on patients with stage I and II tumours.

II.

TADE	Conservative TTT	Radical TTT	Omentectomy + Appendectomy	Peritoneal biopsies	Contralateral ovarian biopsy
I	94,1%	5,9%	17,6%	0%	0%
II	100%	0%	0%	0%	0%

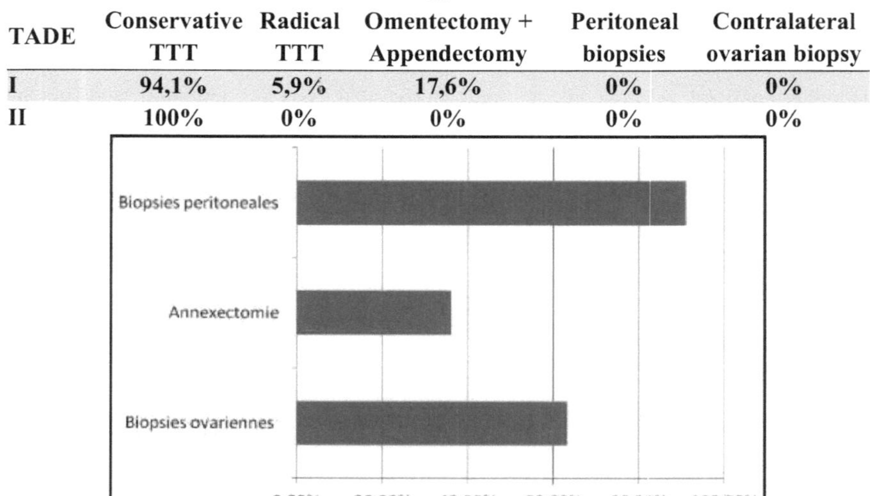

Figure 15: Surgical procedures performed on patients with stage III tumours

V. Histological characteristics of tumours

1. Tumour size

The average tumour size was 150 mm, with extremes ranging from 87 to 270 mm (Figure 16)

Tumour size was greater than 200 mm in 10 cases (33.3%), and less than 200 mm in 20 cases (66.6%). (Figure 17).

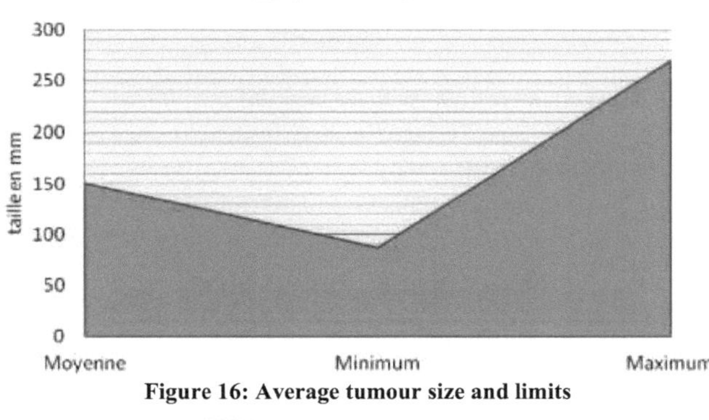

Figure 16: Average tumour size and limits

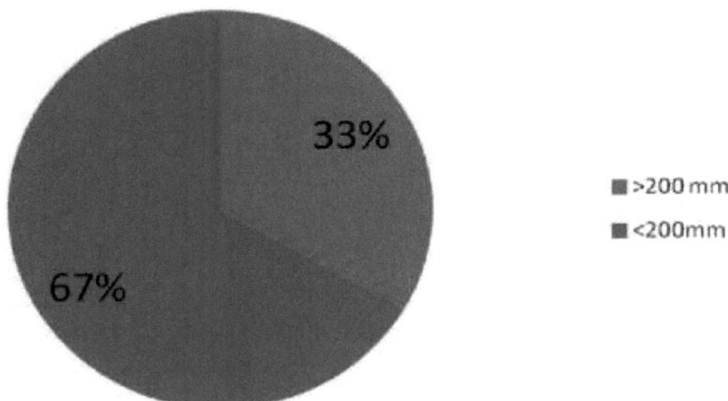

Figure 17: Tumour distribution according to size

2. Lateral lesions

The tumour was located on the right in 15 cases (50%), on the left in 13 cases (40%) and was bilateral in 2 cases, one of which was a dysgerminoma and the second an immature teratoma. (Figure 18)

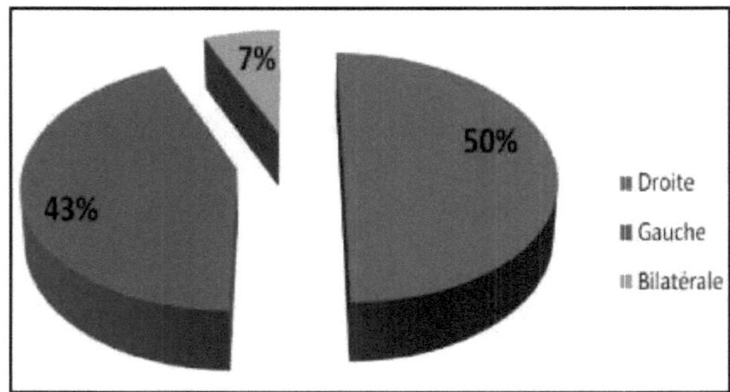

Figure 18: Tumour distribution according to lesion laterality

3. Histological appearance

In agreement with the ultrasound appearance, the tumours were solid-cystic in 18 cases (60%), solid in 9 cases (30%) and purely cystic in 3 cases (Figure 19).

Histological consistency

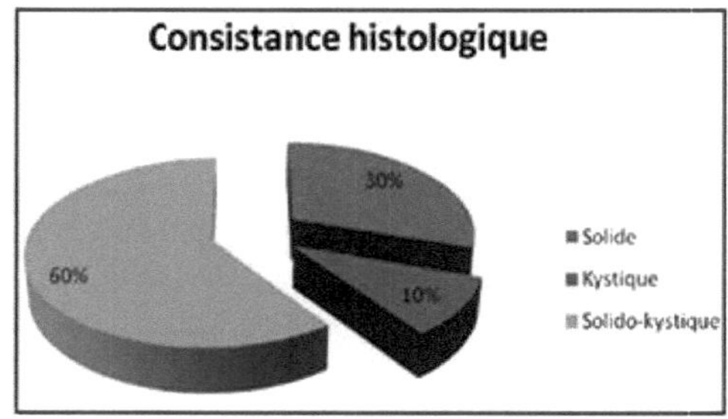

- Solid
- Cystic
- Solid-state

Figure 19: Tumour distribution according to histological appearance

Immature teratomas were solid in 4 cases, solid-cystic in 9 cases and cystic in one case.

The dysgerminomas were purely solid in 5 cases and solid-cystic in 2 cases.

The vitelline tumours were solid-cystic in 2 cases and cystic in one.

Embryonal carcinomas were solid cystic in 4 cases and cystic in one.

The mixed germ cell tumour was solid-cystic.

On histopathological examination, tumour vegetation was present in 67% of cases. (Figure 20).

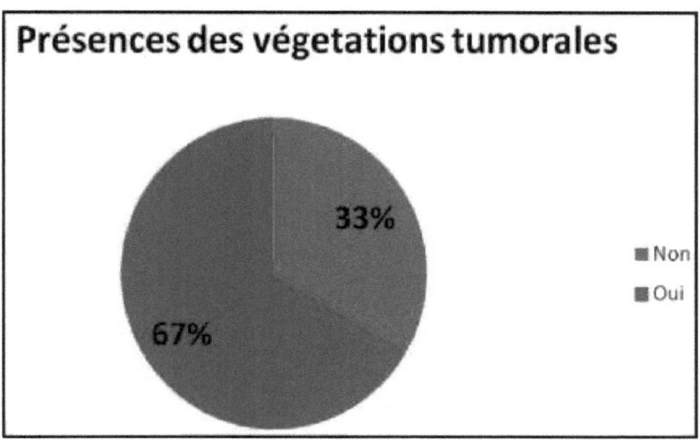

Figure 20: Tumour distribution according to the presence of tumour vegetation

4. Histological types

Our population comprised two main groups:

J Dysgerminomatous tumours or pure dysgerminomas: 7 cases (23%). (Figure 21)

J Non-dysgerminomatous tumours comprising the other histological types of TGMO classes according to the WHO classification, including mixed forms: 23 cases (77%). (Figure 22).

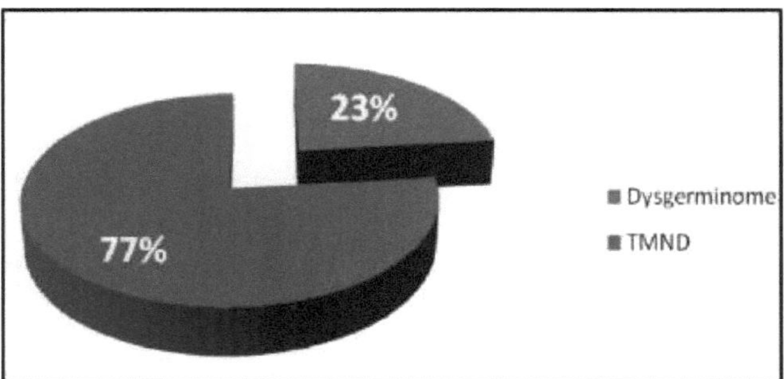

Figure 21: Tumour distribution by histological type

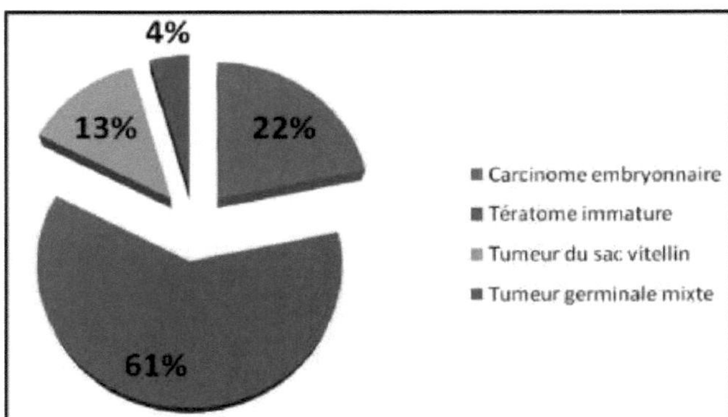

Figure 22: Distribution of TGMND according to hystological type

5. Immunohistochemistry

Immunohistochemical studies were carried out in only 23.3% of cases. (Table IV)
In the 2 cases of vitelline tumours, immunohistochemistry showed intense overexpression of AFP and anticytokeratins.
Overexpression of vimentin and Ki67 was observed in immature teratomas, while immunostaining was negative for EMA, CD20-CD30, E-cadherin, HCG and AFP.
Cytokeratin, EMA, ACE and CD20-CD30 were positive in the 2 cases of embryonal carcinoma, whereas they were negative for dysgerminoma.
(Table IV)

Table IV: Immunohistochemical study of TGMO.

	AFP	Anticytokeratine	Vimentin EMA	PLAP	HCG	CD20/ CD30	ACE
Dysgerminoma	-	-	+	+	+	-	-
Immature teratomas	-	+	++		-	-	
Yolk tumour	++	+	-			-	
Embryonal carcinoma	+	-	++		+	+	+

6. Histological grade

More than half of the immature teratomas were grade 1 (57%) and 37% were grade 2. In our series, only one case of grade 3 immature teratoma was objective. (Figure 23)

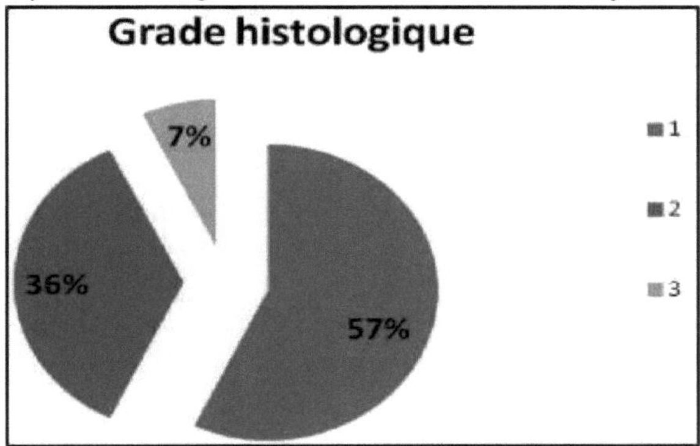

Figure 23: Distribution of immature teratomas by histological grade

7. Histological classification

Patients were classified according to the FIGO classification as follows: (Table V)

Table V: Breakdown of cases according to FIGO classification

Stadium	Number of cases	Percentage
pIA	9	30
pIB	2	6,7
pIC	6	20
pIIA	1	3,3
pIIB	1	3,3
pIIIA	1	3,3
pIIIB	2	6,7
pIIIc	8	26,7
Total	30	100,0

The tumour was classified as stage I and III in 56.7% and 36.7% of cases respectively. Stage IIa represented only 6.7% of cases.
None of the tumours were metastatic.

The distribution of the different histological types according to the FIGO classification is shown in the following table: (Table VI)

Table VI: Histological types according to the FIGO classification.

		Stadium							
		P1A	**GDP**	**PIC**	**PИA**	**PUB**	**PIIIA**	**PIIIB**	**PIIIC**
Carcinoma embryonic	**Workforce**	**0**	**0**	**0**	**0**	**0**	**0**	**1**	**4**
	%	**0,0%**	**0,0%**	**0,0%**	**0,0%**	**0,0%**	**0,0%**	**20%**	**80%**
Dysgerminoma	**Workforce**	**1**	**1**	**2**	**1**	**0**	**0**	**0**	**2**
	%	**14,3%**	**14,3%**	**28,6%**	**14,3%**	**0,0%**	**0,0%**	**0,0%**	**28,6%**
Immature teratoma	**Workforce**	**8**	**1**	**3**	**0**	**0**	**1**	**0**	**1**
	%	**57,1%**	**7,1%**	**21,4%**	**0,0%**	**0,0%**	**7,1%**	**0,0%**	**7,1%**
Bag tumour vitellin	**Workforce**	**0**	**0**	**1**	**0**	**1**	**0**	**0**	**1**
	%	**0,0%**	**0,0%**	**33,3%**	**0,0%**	**33,3%**	**0,0%**	**0,0%**	**33,3%**
Germ cell tumour mixed	**Workforce**	**0**	**0**	**0**	**0**	**0**	**0**	**1**	**0**
	%	**0,0%**	**0,0%**	**0,0%**	**0,0%**	**0,0%**	**0,0%**	**100%**	**0,0%**
Total	**Workforce**	**9**	**2**	**6**	**1**	**1**	**1**	**2**	**8**
	%	**30%**	**6,7%**	**20%**	**3,3%**	**3,3%**	**3,3%**	**6,7%**	**26,7%**

Stage I was observed in 4 cases of dysgerminoma (23.5%) and 13 cases of TGMND (76.4%), while stage III was observed in 2 cases of dysgerminoma (18.1%) and 9 cases of TGMND (81.8%).

Stage I was most frequently observed in immature teratomas.

Stage III was most frequently observed in embryonal carcinomas.

VI. Therapeutic management

1. Surgical treatment

Surgical treatment was radical in 07 patients (23.3%) and conservative leaving an ovary and uterus in place in 23 patients (76.7%). (Table XII)

Table VII: Type of surgery according to FIGO stages.

	TREATMENT			
	Radical		**Curator**	**Total**
Workforce PlA	**1**	**8**		**9**
%	**11,1%**	**88,9%**		**100%**
GDP headcount	**1**	**1**		**2**
%	**50%**			**50%100%**
PIC workforce	**2**	**4**		**6**
%	**33,3%**	**66,7%**		**100%**
Workforce PIIA	**0**	**1**		**1**
%	**0,0%**	**100%**		**100%**
Headcount PIIB	**0**	**1**		**1**
%	**0,0%**	**100%**		**100%**
Headcount PIIIA	**0**	**1**		**1**
%	**0,0%**	**100%**		**100%**
Workforce PIIIB	**1**	**1**		**2**
%	**50%**			**50%100%**
Headcount PIIIC	**2**	**6**		**8**
%	**25%**		**75%**	**100%**

Workforce Total	**7**	**23**	**30**
%	23,3%	76,7%	**100%**

In the group of patients with early-stage OMT, repeat surgery was performed for staging and for surgical totalization in 3 patients who had already had their number of children:

- ❖ One had a cystectomy alone (stage IA),
- ❖ The second had a unilateral adnexectomy and contralateral lumpectomy for a tumour classified IB.
- ❖ The third had a unilateral adnexectomy for an IC class tumour and was 40 years old.

Among patients with advanced BMD, radical surgery was performed in 3 cases:

- ❖ one of them underwent neoadjuvant chemotherapy for a stage IIIC mixed germ cell tumour with an incomplete response (tumour reduction estimated at 50% with negative tumour markers); surgery was complete with no tumour residue but pelvic and lumbo-aortic lymph node dissection was positive.
- ❖ The other two were stage IIIC dysgerminomas having undergone neoadjuvant chemotherapy with a complete response in one case and a partial response in the other. Surgery was not complete in the latter case.

Lymph node dissection was carried out in these two patients and was positive in one. All these procedures were performed laparotomically.

2. Chemotherapy

Of the cases consulted, six patients did not receive adjuvant chemotherapy and rigorous monitoring was recommended in 4.

Complementary treatment to surgery in the form of polychemotherapy was indicated in 14 patients (46.6%), while 10 patients (33.3%) received neoadjuvant chemotherapy (Figure 24).

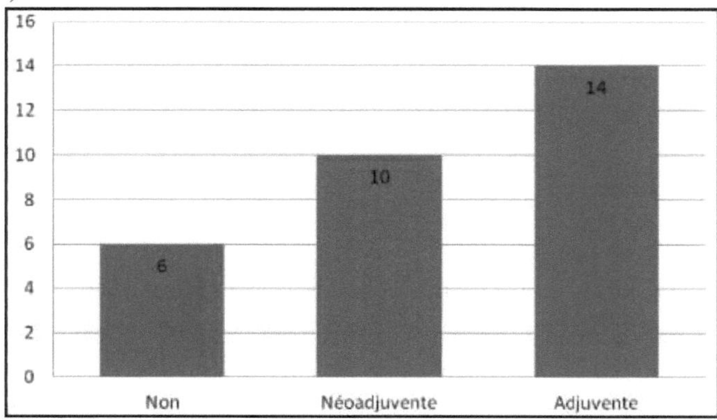

Figure 24: Distribution of patients according to complementary treatment

2.1. Protocols, number of courses and administration times

Platinum-based chemotherapy was used in 100% of cases.

The BEP (Bleomycin- Etoposide- Cisplatin) protocol was used in 21 cases, BVP (Bleomycin- Vinblastine- Cisplatin) in 2 patients and VIP (Etoposide + Ifosfamide + cisPlatin) in one patient. (Figure 25)

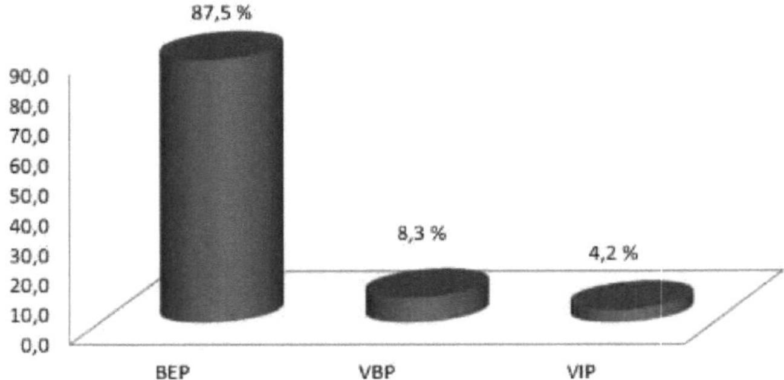

Figure 25: The different chemotherapy protocols

The number of courses of treatment ranged from 2 to 5. (Figure 26).

Chemotherapy was started on average 29 days after the initial surgical treatment, with extremes ranging from 10 to 90 days.

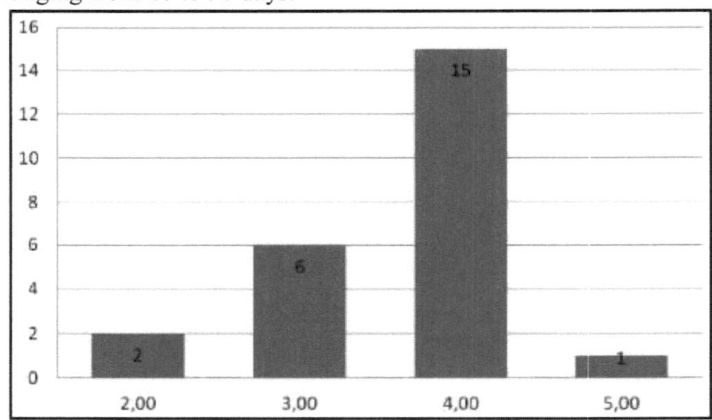

Figure 26: Distribution of patients according to the number of courses of chemotherapy.

2.2. Indications

Adjuvant chemotherapy was indicated in 3 cases of dysgerminoma (21.4%), 2 of which were stage IC and one stage IIA.

Adjuvant chemotherapy was indicated for TGMND in 78.5% of cases:

J 9 cases of immature teratoma, 5 of which were stage IA, one stage IB and 3 stage IC.

J 2 cases of yolk tumour: one stage IC and one stage IIB (Table VIII)

Table VIII: Adjuvant chemotherapy according to stage and histological type.

tade	Histological type	Type of chemotherapy	Protoc ole	No.
IA	Immature teratoma	Adjuvant	BEP	3
IA	Immature teratoma	Adjuvant	BEP	3

IA	Immature teratoma	Adjuvant	BEP	4
IA	Immature teratoma	Adjuvant	BEP	4
IA	Immature teratoma	Adjuvant	BEP	4
IB	Immature teratoma	Adjuvant	BEP	4
IC	Immature teratoma	Adjuvant	BEP	4
IC	Immature teratoma	Adjuvant	BEP	4
IC	Immature teratoma	Adjuvant	BEP	4
IC	Dysgerminoma	Adjuvant	BEP	4
IC	Dysgerminoma	Adjuvant	BEP	4
IC	Yolk sac tumour	Adjuvant	BEP	4
IIA	Dysgerminoma	Adjuvant	VBP	3
IIB	Vitelline Sac Tumour	Adjuvant	BEP	4

Neoadjuvant chemotherapy was indicated for all stage III tumours (Table IX).

Table IX: Neoadjuvant chemotherapy according to stage and histological type.

Stadium	Histological type	Type of chemotherapy	Protocol	No.
IIIB	Mixed germ cell tumour	Neoadjuvant	VIP	5
IIIB	Embryonal carcinoma	Neoadjuvant	VBP	4
IIIC	Embryonal carcinoma	Neoadjuvant	BEP	3
IIIC	Embryonal carcinoma	Neoadjuvant	BEP	2
IIIC	Embryonal carcinoma	Neoadjuvant	BEP	4
IIIC	Embryonal carcinoma	Neoadjuvant	BEP	3
IIIC	Dysgerminoma	Neoadjuvant	BEP	4
IIIC	Dysgerminoma	Neoadjuvant	BEP	4
IIIC	Immature teratoma	Neoadjuvant	BEP	3
IIIC	Yolk sac tumour	Neoadjuvant	BEP	2

2.3. Complications

Complications of chemotherapy were observed in 4 patients (16.66%) and included :

- Hematological toxicity in two patients, with anemia and neutropenia.
- Bleomycin-induced pneumonitis in a patient.
- Renal failure in one patient.

3. Radiotherapy

Radiotherapy was performed on a single 10-year-old prepubertal girl and the field of irradiation was the lumbo-aortic lymph nodes.

VI. Evolution

In our series, a patient with incomplete post-chemotherapy resection of a stage IIIC dysgerminoma was reported to continue to progress. This patient had developed hepatic metastasis, and second-line chemotherapy was initiated.

We observed 3 cases of metastatic recurrence, which occurred after an average period of 48 months, with extremes ranging from 24 to 120 months.

The two cases of recurrence were observed in patients who had not received adjuvant treatment and had escaped: the first case was a stage IA grade III immature teratoma, and the second was a stage IIIA.

The third recurrence was in the metastatic form of a stage IIIB mixed germ cell tumour which had undergone radical surgery with pelvic and lumbo-aortic curage.
The metastases were located in the liver in one patient, in the lung in the second, and in the mediastinum and supra-clavicular lymph nodes in the other two.
Treatment consisted of chemotherapy in all cases. (Table X)

Table X: Recurrence and metastasis according to histological type.

		Recurrence/ Metastasis	
		No	**Yes**
PIA	Workforce	8	1
	%	88,9%	11,1%
GDP	Workforce	2	0
	%	100,0%	0,0%
PIC	Workforce	6	0
	%	100,0%	0,0%
PDA	Workforce	1	0
	%	100,0%	0,0%
PIIB	Workforce	1	0
	%	100,0%	0,0%
PIIIA	Workforce	0	1
	%	0,0%	100,0%
PIIIB	Workforce	1	1
	%	50,0%	50,0%
PIIIC	Workforce	7	1
	%	87,5%	12,5%

VII. Survival

1. Overall survival

Survival was studied in our series for all patients.
The development date was October 2019 and we consulted our patients in December 2019 by telephone.
Two patients were lost to follow-up after 4 and 6 years.
Of the 28 patients, 21 were in complete remission, i.e. 75% of cases.
There were 7 cases of death between 12 months and 180 months after surgery.
The cause of death was unrelated to the disease in one case: a vitelline IIIc tumour that died of an unknown cause 48 months after conservative treatment followed by only 2 courses of chemotherapy.
Death was related to the disease in the remaining 6 patients. In these patients, the tumour was classified as stage IA, stage IIIA, stage III B and stage IIIC in 3 cases. (Table XI)
The first three cases of death occurred 12 months, 45 months and 48 months after the positive diagnosis of cancer.

Table XI: Death according to histological type, stage and therapeutic options.

Stadium	Histological type	Surgical treatment	Chemotherapy	Type	number	Deaths	Survival (months)
IA	TERATOME	CONSERVATO	NO			YES	60

	IMMATURE	R				
IIIA	TERATOME IMMATURE	CONSERVATOR	NO		YES	45
IIIB	GERM CELL TUMOUR MIXED	RADICAL	NEOADJUVENTE	VIP 5	YES	120
IIIC	CARCINOME EMBRYONARY	CONSERVATOR	NEOADJUVENTE	BEP 2	YES	180
IIIC	DYSGERMINOME	RADICAL	NEOADJUVENTE	BEP 4	YES	90
IIIC	BAG TUMOR VITELIN	CONSERVATOR	NEOADJUVENTE	BEP 2	YES	48
IIIC	DYSGERMINOME	RADICAL	NEOADJUVENTE	BEP 4	YES	12

In our series, the average survival of the population studied was 94 months, with extremes ranging from 1 to 250 months.

Overall survival for all stages was 96.7% at 2 years, 85.7% at 5 years and 75.8% at 10 years.

Overall survival at 20 years was 56.4%. (Figure 27)

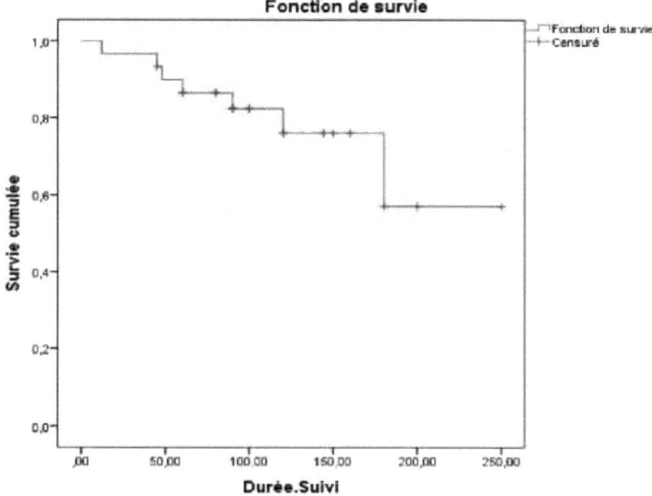

Figure 27: Overall survival

2. Survival as a function of age

Age was a significant prognostic factor (P=0.011). (Figure 28)

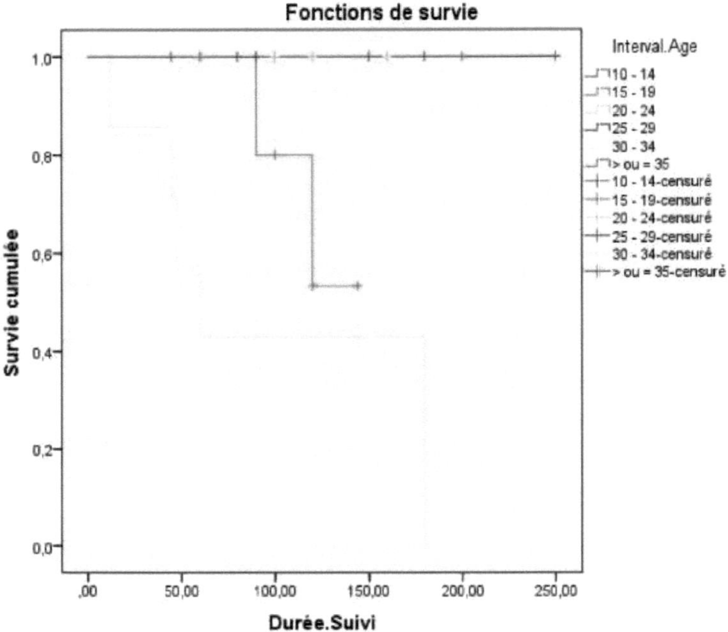

Figure 28: Overall survival by age group

Overall survival for patients over 30 years of age was 50%, whereas for women under 30 years of age it was 90%. This difference was statistically significant (P=0.029). Overall survival at 2 and 5 years was better in patients aged under 30. It was 100%. For patients aged over 30, survival was 85% at 5 years and 68% at 5 years. This difference was also statistically significant (P=0.029). (Figure 29)

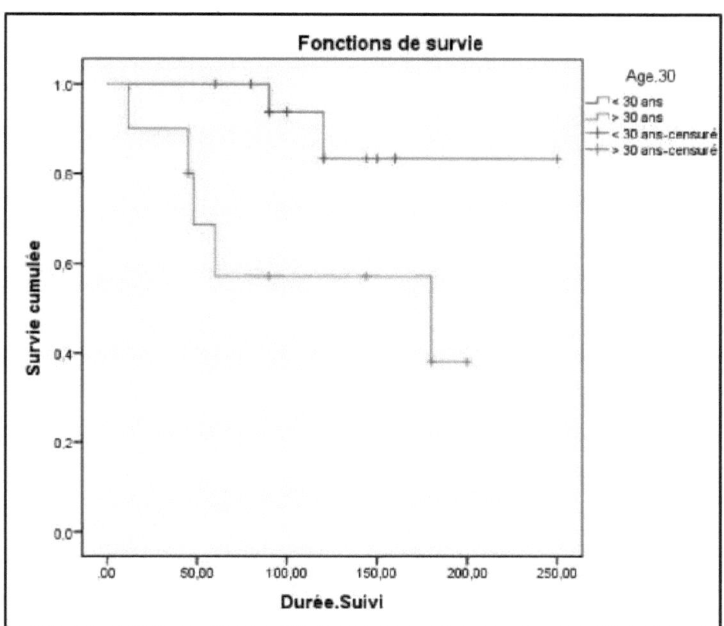

Figure 29: Overall survival as a function of Page

3. Survival as a function of tumour size

Overall survival for patients with tumours <20 cm in size was better than those with tumours >20 cm in size.

In fact, for tumours >20 cm in size, survival at 5 and 10 years was 60%, and for those <20 cm in size, it was 100% at 5 years (P = 0.004) (Figure 30).

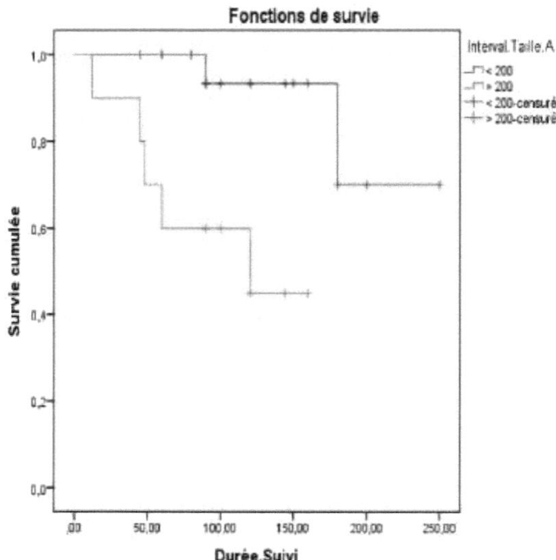

Figure 30: Overall survival as a function of tumour size

4. Survival according to tumour stage

Overall survival at 5 and 10 years for patients classified as stage I was 94.7%.
The rate for patients classified as stage II was 100%.
In patients classified as stage III, overall survival at 5 years was 73.2% and 62.4% respectively. (Figure 31/32)
The difference was statistically significant (P=0.014).

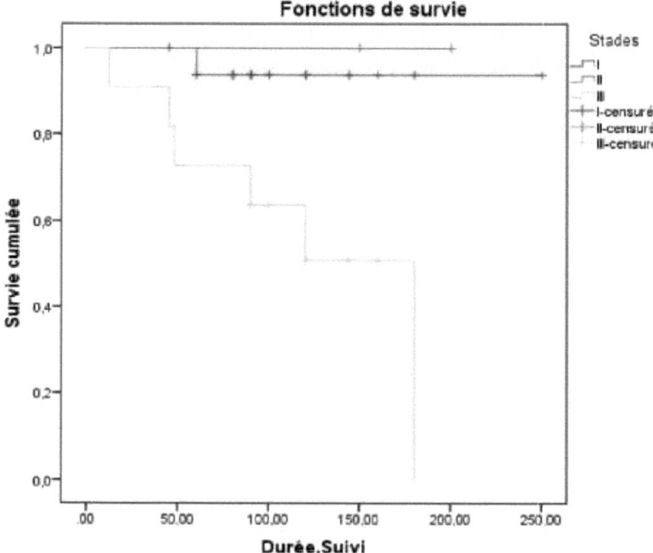

Figure 31: Overall survival as a function of tumour stage

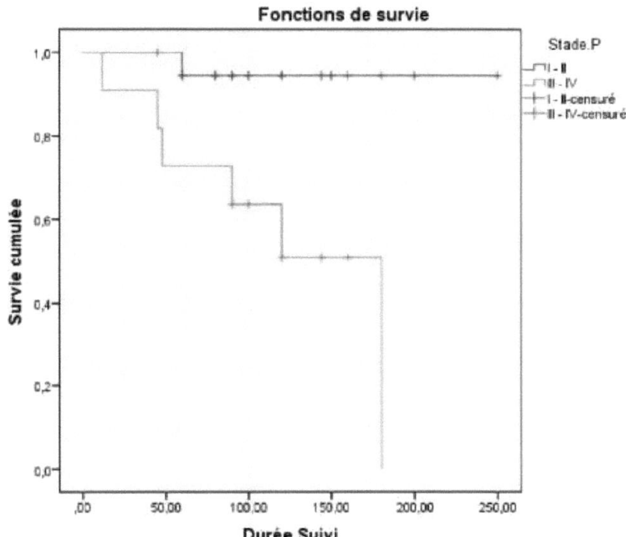

Figure 32: Overall survival according to combined tumour stage

5. Survival as a function of consultation time

Overall survival was better for patients who consulted before the 6th month of evolution; it was 86.4%, whereas for women who consulted after an interval of 6 months it was 50%. This difference was statistically significant (P=0.033). (Figure 33)

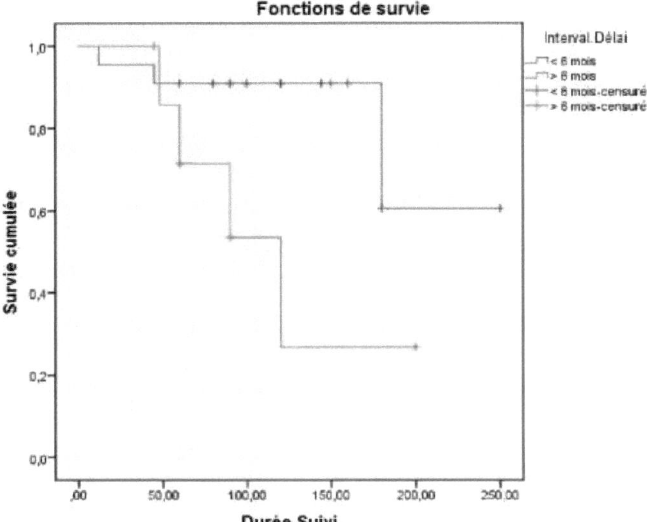

Figure 33: Survival as a function of consultation time

6. Survival according to histological type

Overall survival was better for non-dysgerminomatous BMSCT than for dysgerminomatous BMSCT at 2 and 10 years. This difference was not statistically significant (P=0.053). (Figure 34)

Overall survival was slightly better for immature teratomas than for other TNMNDs. It was 85.7%, 80% for embryonal carcinomas and 66.7% for vitelline tumours (P = 0.054) (Figure 35).

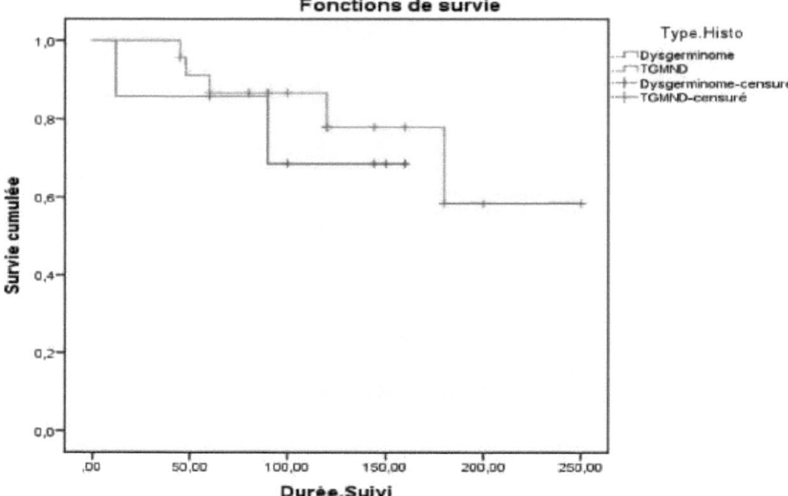

Figure 34: Survival by histological type

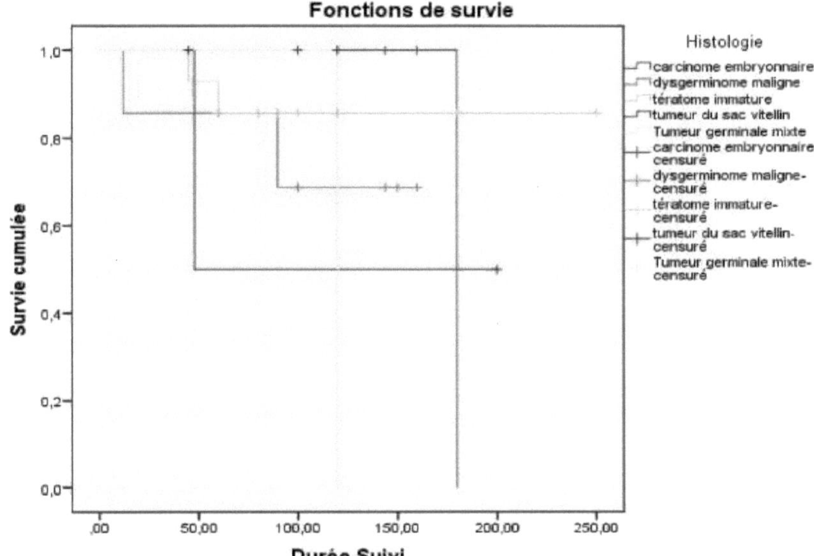

Figure 35: Survival by histological subtype

7. Survival according to type of surgery

Short-term overall survival (2 and 5 years) was comparable between patients with conservative and radical treatment.

However, in the long term (10 years), it was better in patients who had undergone conservative treatment: 83% versus 50%.

This difference was not statistically significant (P=0.34). (Figure 36).

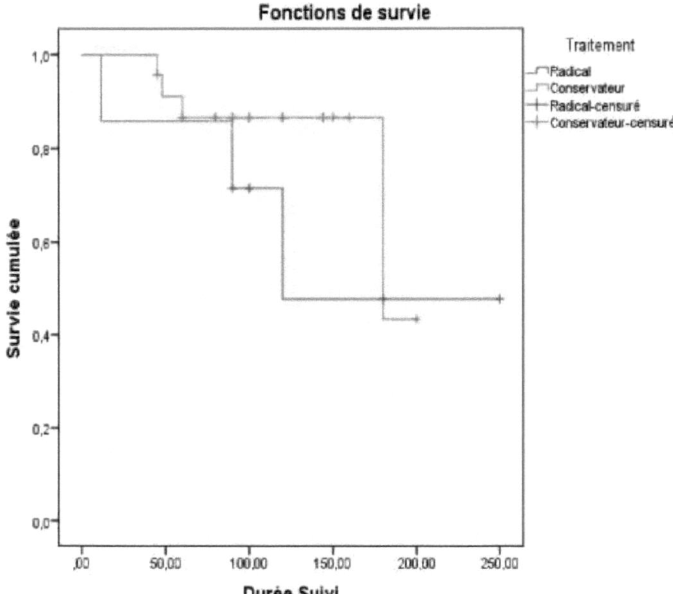

Figure 36: Survival by type of surgery

8. Survival according to histological grade

There was no significant difference between the three histological grades for immature teratomas in terms of overall survival (P=0.13) (Figure 37).

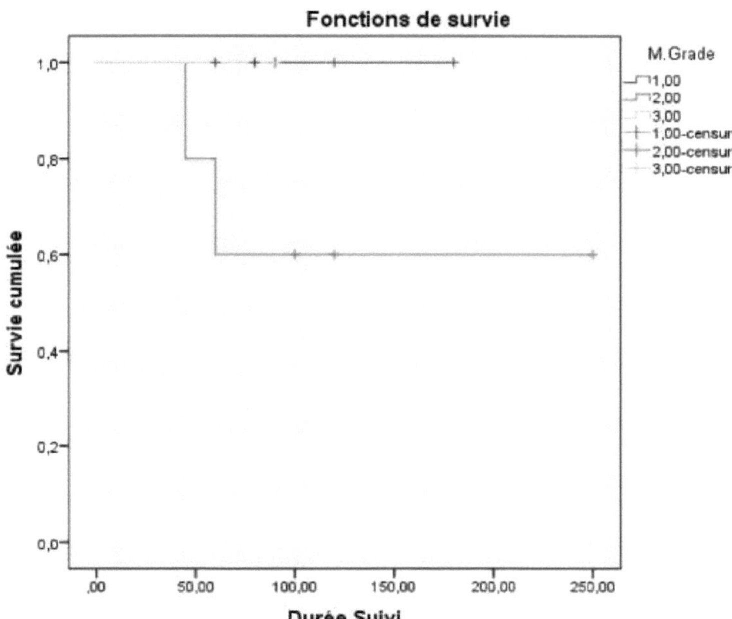

Figure 37: Overall survival of immature teratomas according to histological grade

9. Survival as a function of the number of courses of chemotherapy

Overall survival was better in patients receiving three or four courses of chemotherapy compared with those receiving only two courses. (P= 0,57)
(Figure 38)

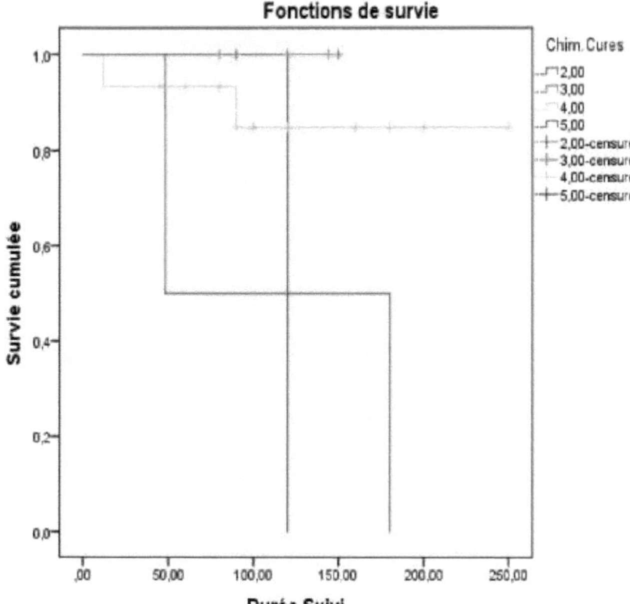

Figure 38: Survival as a function of number of courses of chemotherapy

VIII. Fertility

Of the 17 patients who had previously undergone conservative treatment, 9 achieved pregnancy, 7 of them spontaneously and 2 induced (for male infertility).

Of the other seven patients, 5 are still single and unmarried, 2 already had children and are currently on a levonorgestrel intrauterine device (IUD).

4 Discussion

A. Discussion of the methodology

Our study is a retrospective descriptive study carried out in the Gynecology-Obstetrics, Medical Oncology and Anatomopathology Departments of the FARHAT HACHED University Hospital in Sousse over a period of 21 years (1st September 1998 to 30th September 2019). This work made it possible to collect the various clinical, histological and therapeutical data of a rather rare ovarian pathology which is the malignant germinal pathology of the ovary (TGMO).

In the course of this work, we used a data collection form which, in addition to epidemiological data, included clinical, radiological, biological, anatomopathological, therapeutic and prognostic data.

The sample size is 30 patients with GIST. It would be interesting to carry out the study on a larger series, but given that the pathology in question is very rare, a prospective study seems difficult and not feasible. Nevertheless, this is the largest Tunisian series relating to TGMO.

Although the size of this study is small, the results appear to be consistent with larger series. However, it would be more interesting to collect the other cases of TGMO diagnosed at the level of the other cancer registries in the country in order to establish a national series of this tumour, within the framework of a national registry of rare ovarian tumours as is the case in other European countries.

The data was collected from medical records and the information may sometimes be missing or incomplete.

The use of telephone data collection relatively alters the accuracy of the information.

The study poses the problem of the heterogeneity of the study population in terms of age, desire for pregnancy and genital activity. On the other hand, it enables the disease to be studied in two distinct groups, and subsequently two possible strategies adapted to the prognosis of this pathological entity to be established.

B. Discussion of results

The aims of our study were to describe the epidemiological, diagnostic, anatomopathological, therapeutic and prognostic features of malignant germ cell tumours of the ovary in the Gynecology-Obstetrics Department of the FARHAT HACHED University Hospital in Sousse, and to compare our results with the literature in order to propose a decisional diagram that could improve the management of this entity in our context.

I. Epidemiological data

1. Frequency

GISTs are rare gynaecological neoplasms. They represent approximately 2% to 3% of all ovarian cancers in Western countries and 29% of all malignant germ cell tumours. [9]

It occurs mainly in young women, with an incidence rate of 75% in women aged under 30 [9].

In 2011, the number of new cases worldwide was 5.3 per million. [10] In most countries, the rate of occurrence is on average less than 3% of the population. [11] However, Asia reported the highest proportion of cases at 4.3% due to the younger age profile of the population. [11] For the other regions, the reported incidence rates are 2.5% in Oceania, 2.0% in North America and 1.3% in Europe. [11]

Among other things, ethnic and racial differences have been noted, with an increased incidence of TGMO in black and oriental women, who present 5 to 14% of ovarian cancers, in contrast to western women, where they represent 2% of ovarian cancers. [12]

In our series, the incidence of TGMO was 4.7%. We are in line with these studies.

1.1. Dysgerminomas

Dysgerminomas are comparable to testicular seminomas. It is the most common histological variant of OMGTs and accounts for 40% of malignant germ cell tumours of the ovary. [13]

However, dysgerminomas occur less frequently in black women. In fact, in a study including 2196 patients with BMT, 1654 of whom were Caucasian and 328 Black, the author reported that 28.5% of tumours were dysgerminomas and that the frequency of the latter was higher in Caucasian patients (32.9% vs 9.8% in Black women). [12]

In our study, their frequency was 23%.

1.2. TGMND

The Surveillance, Epidemiology and End Results Registry (SEER) of the National Cancer Institute reported that immature teratomas were the most common form of TGMND accounting for 35.6%, followed by yolk sac tumours (14.4%), and less frequently mixed germ cell tumours (5.3%) and embryonal carcinoma (4.1%) [14]. These results were similar to those of Hinchcliff et al, who also showed that immature teratomas occurred less frequently in white women (35.5%) compared with black women (50%) [12].

Table XII: TGMND frequencies

	SEER / National Cancer Institute	Our results
Immature teratoma	**35,6%**	**46.7%**
Yolk sac tumour	**14,4%**	**10%**
Embryonal carcinoma	**4,1%**	**16,7%**
Mixed germ cell tumours	**5,3%**	**3.3%**

Choriocarcinomas are exceptionally rare and represent 2.1% to 3.4% of all TGMOs. [14]

Reviewing the literature, choriocarcinomas are rarer in their pure form, and are often associated with other contingents such as immature teratomas, dysgerminomas and embryonal carcinomas, because their embryological origin is identical. [15]

We found no cases of pure or impure choriocarcinoma in our series.

In our study, contrary to what had been previously reported by several authors, the immature teratoma was the most frequently represented type of TGMO (46.7%).

2. Age of onset

According to the literature, the incidence of ovarian cancer is 0.1 per 100,000 women in girls under the age of 9, compared with 1.1 per 100,000 in girls aged 10-19, with the majority (~80%) being TGMO in all age groups [16].

GVHD may be present in early childhood, but its incidence rises sharply from the age of 5 and continues with the onset of puberty, reaching a peak incidence rate of 1.2 per 100,000 women aged 15 to 19 [17 - 18].

The most common histological subtype in these young girls is dysgerminoma [18]. Most of these occur before the age of 40, with 75% diagnosed between the ages of 10 and 30, whereas immature teratomas are usually diagnosed around the age of 20, and ovarian yolk sac tumours and embryonal carcinomas are diagnosed before the patient reaches the age of 20 [19].

A few rare publications have described the occurrence of TGMO in patients aged over 50. [20]

In our series, the mean age of patients with immature teratomas was 25 years, while that of patients with embryonal carcinomas and endodermal sinus tumours was 21 and 35 years respectively.

3. Risk factors

Despite the multitude of studies carried out in an attempt to identify the etiological factors responsible for the genesis of TGMO, the exact cause of TGMO remains to be determined.

3.1. Genetic factor

The existence of familial cases and the young age at onset of GIST suggest the existence of a hereditary genetic predisposition or cause. This hypothesis has been underlined by a number of epidemiological studies which have shown that genetic alterations can contribute to the development of GISTs, such as classical tumour suppressor genes and oncogenes.

According to I. Ray-Coquard, GISTs are linked to the presence of an iso chromosome on the short arm of chromosome 12, [i (12p)], which is not found in any other type of cancer. [21] while mutation of the C-Kit gene encoding the tyrosine kinase receptor has an important role in seminomatous differentiation according to Tian Q. [22]

On the other hand, individuals with autosomal BRCA-1 / BRCA-2 mutations are generally more prone to develop TGMO. [23]

Families with TGMO are rare. To date, only 10 families have been reported with both testicular and ovarian germ cell malignancies and 8 families with 2 family members with TGMO [24].

In most of these families, pure dysgerminoma is the most common tumour, followed by immature teratoma and mixed germ cell tumours. [24]

In our series, there were no familial cases of TGMO.

3.2. Gonadal dysgenesis

The role of gonadal dysgenesis has also been suggested by many authors, given its

frequent association with TGMO [25, 26]. In the series by RZEPKA et al. 10.1% of patients had gonadal dysgenesis and an abnormal karyotype [25].
Gonadoblastomas, which are benign tumours arising almost exclusively in dysgenic gonads, and which in 50% of cases progress to BMT, have been given the name germ cell tumour in situ [26, 27, 28].

3.3. Other factors

Nowadays, a number of risk factors have been identified, including endometriosis, polycystic ovary syndrome, hormonal exposure and maternal use of exogenous hormones (oral contraception after conception), high maternal body mass index and an age at first pregnancy of less than 20 years [23].
In addition to genetic modifications, environmental factors such as exposure to hazardous substances, including plastics, pesticides and dioxins, may also contribute to the proliferation of BMTs. [23]
For Schulman LP, interactions between germline and somatic mutations on the one hand, and environmental factors on the other, could be responsible for the phenotypic expression of TGMOs. [29]
Regarding immature teratomas, the literature review did not find any risk factors apart from the fact that these are generally young nulligravida patients who may have a history of dermoid cysts. [30]
In our series, young age and nulligestion are the main risk factors.
None of our patients presented symptoms that could correspond to gonadal dysgenesis (delayed puberty and/or delayed height and weight), but one patient had previously undergone surgery for a mature teratoma.

II. CLINICAL STUDY Clinical study

1. Circumstances of discovery

Today, there are no pathognomonic symptoms or signs for GIST, and these signs are often multiple, subtle and non-specific.
According to the majority of authors, abdominal pain associated with a palpable pelvic-abdominal mass remains the major symptom and is present in approximately 85% of patients. [31]
Acute abdominal pain' , due to adnexal torsion or tumour rupture, may be experienced in rare cases and may present as an acute abdominal syndrome. Indeed, endodermal sinus tumours or tumours with a mixed component are often misdiagnosed as acute appendicitis because of their acute presentation. [31]
Other less common signs are abdominal distension (35%), fever (10%), ascites (10%) and vaginal bleeding (10%) [32].
More rarely, it is the finding and appearance of a critical indicator of malignancy: the "Mary Joseph sreur" nodule, which may lead to the diagnosis. [33]
In our series, abdominal enlargement was observed in 17% of patients and abdominal pain in 45%.
The acute abdominal symptomatology was present in a patient undergoing emergency surgery for suspected adnexal torsion and was a twisted stage IA dysgerminoma.

These tumours may be discovered incidentally; in 37% of dysgerminomas according to ABOUT, 20% of immature teratomas according to HESLAN [34, 30]. In one of our patients, the discovery was fortuitous during investigation of thrombophlebitis.
Altered general condition was observed in 25% of cases in ABOUT's series [34] and in 11% of cases in our study. Fever was present in 10-25% of cases [35].
It is also important to note the frequency of the association of TGMO and pregnancy which can reach 25 to 35% of dysgerminomas whereas it is only 2 to 5% for all malignant tumours of the ovary, this frequency being explained by the occurrence of these tumours in patients of childbearing age. [36, 37]
In our series, no cases of pregnancy were observed.

2. Consultation deadline

There are major clinical differences between GIST and epithelial ovarian carcinoma. Ovarian epithelial carcinoma remains silent for a long time, whereas GIST progresses rapidly and symptoms often develop and appear within a short time. This explains why GIST is often diagnosed when the disease is still at an early stage.
TGMOs can grow very rapidly. Kurman and Norris [38], in their series of 71 cases of ovarian yolk sac tumour, described the case of two patients who had normal examinations 4 weeks before the discovery of their tumours (9 cm and 12 cm larger diameter). They also described another case of a woman who had been monitored at regular intervals since the start of her pregnancy and who developed a 23 cm tumour at the time of her oophorectomy (performed at 14 weeks' gestation). This rapid growth rate may explain the high rate of capsular tears observed at surgery and on pathological examination.
In our series, the average time between the appearance of the first signs and the date of consultation was 3 months. For stage III, it was 4.5 months, while for stage I it was 3 months.

III. RADIOLOGICAL INVESTIGATIONS Radiological investigations

1. Pelvic ultrasound

This is the key paraclinical examination for exploring adnexal masses and ovarian tumours in particular. It points to the organic nature of the tumour and allows a presumption of malignancy to be established by morphological analysis of the ovarian tumour, and by demonstration of ascites, pelvic adenopathy and/or hepatic or peritoneal metastases.
For Emoto et al, the use of ultrasound combined with colour Doppler via the trans-vaginal route makes it possible to differentiate between benign and malignant tumours by assessing intra-tumoral blood flow. [39]

2. Abdominal and pelvic CT scan

Computed tomography (CT) is not always necessary for diagnosis; it is a non-compulsory adjunct to ultrasound for diagnosis and for establishing the extent of ovarian tumours.
It allows an abdomino-pelvic mass to be attached to the ovary.

CT is not the best way of exploring small tumours, but it remains essential for preoperative extension assessment, postoperative surveillance and early diagnosis of recurrence.

Abdominal and pelvic CT scans can also be used to explore lymph node areas.

3. Magnetic resonance imaging (MRI)

It is playing an increasingly important role in the investigation of pelvic tumours. Its tissue sensitivity allows perfect anatomical delineation and more detailed characterisation of the lesion, which is particularly important when there is a dysgerminomatous component. [40]

Magnetic resonance imaging can be used to establish the origin of pelvic tumours and their relationship with neighbouring organs (bladder, rectum) and the pelvis.

pelvic wall. It therefore has a dual role: to establish the locoregional extension and to monitor treated tumours.

In our series, ultrasound was performed in 24 (80%) of our patients. It showed an adnexal mass with a heterogeneous echo structure in 87.5% of cases, with a solid cystic appearance in 66.7% of cases, and revealed ascites in 37.5% of cases.

CT scans were carried out in 11 of our patients, confirming the ultrasound findings and enabling the mass to be associated with the ovary in the two cases where the tumour origin could not be determined by ultrasound.

100% of patients who received a CT scan had a tumour formation >150mm. There was no lymph node involvement on abdominopelvic CT.

4.1. Radiological aspects of dysgerminomas

With a few exceptions, dysgerminomas are typically purely solid. On ultrasound, they are divided into lobules, with heterogeneous echogenicity, smooth lobular contours and well-defined borders, and are richly vascularised on colour Doppler. [41]

The lobular appearance is also seen on CT scan; the tumour is predominantly solid, with patches of necrosis separated by vascularised septa. Calcifications may be present in a speckled appearance. [41]

The most characteristic image on magnetic resonance imaging (MRI) is that of a solid mass divided into lobules by fibro-vascular septa. Dysgerminomas have low signal intensity relative to muscle on T1-weighted images and are isointense or slightly hyperintense on T2-weighted images. Usually, septa are hypointense or isointense on T2-weighted images and difficult to appreciate on T1-weighted images, with intense enhancement after contrast administration. [41]

4.2. Radiological aspects of yolk sac tumours

Imaging findings of yolk sac tumours often include a mixed solid and cystic mass with a hemorrhagic component. The external contour is generally smooth [41].

On ultrasound, the solid components are heterogeneously echogenic and the cystic spaces are divided by septa.

The bright spot sign is a common finding on MRI and CT. These foci of enhancement are attributed to dilated vessels, given the highly vascular nature of these tumours. Although common, the light spot sign is not pathognomonic for yolk sac tumour as other germ cell tumours may have similar morphological features. [41].

Another imaging feature described in yolk sac tumours is capsular tears. Although commonly seen in yolk sac tumours, capsular tears are not pathognomonic as other ovarian tumours, including mature cystic teratomas, may present with capsular tears [41]. Areas of hemorrhage have a high signal intensity on T1-weighted MRI images.

4.3. Radiological aspects of immature teratomas

Imaging of immature teratomas is non-specific and resembles other solid ovarian neoplasia on ultrasound, appearing as a heterogeneous solid mass with small scattered calcifications. Foci of fat appear as areas of increased echogenicity [41].

On MRI and CT, immature teratomas appear as a predominantly solid mass with coarse irregular calcifications and numerous cysts of variable size. The solid component has soft tissue attenuation on CT and a wide range of signal intensities on T2-weighted imaging.

Unlike mature cystic teratomas, in which the cysts predominantly contain fatty sebaceous fluid, in immature teratomas the cysts predominantly have an attenuation and signal intensity similar to that of plain fluid [41] and in immature teratomas the calcifications are small, irregular and scattered throughout the tumour, whereas in mature cystic teratomas they are generally coarse or tooth-shaped.

4.4. Radiological aspects of non-gestational choriocarcinomas

Few reports are available on the imaging features of non-gestational choriocarcinoma. However, a well-defined adnexal mass of mixed echogenicity on pelvic ultrasound has been described. This helps to exclude uterine or extra-uterine pregnancy in patients with high levels of eHCG.

On MRI, abnormal signal attenuations representing vascular structures and small cystic cavities are seen in solid components on T2-weighted imaging, and foci with high signal intensity, resulting from hemorrhage, can be seen in solid parts on T1-weighted imaging [41].

5. Radiological aspects of mixed germ cell tumours

To our knowledge, there are no reports on the radiological features of mixed GISTs. In our experience, they manifest as a solid mass with areas of cystic change resulting from hemorrhage or necrosis or a cystic lesion with solid components. Intra-lesional fat or calcifications may be seen if an immature teratoma element is present.

IV. Tumour markers

Tumour markers have multiple benefits, both at the diagnostic and therapeutic stages and during subsequent follow-up. [42]

TGMOs can secrete four biological markers which differ according to the histological type of tumour: gonadotropic chorionic hormone (HCG), the free beta subunit of this hormone (eHCG), alpha-freeto-proteine (AFP) and lactate dehydrogenase (LDH). [42]

TGMO can be associated with an increase in alkaline phosphatase and cancer antigen 125. [43]

These tumour markers can be found either in situ by immunohistochemical methods, or in the circulating state in plasma. [43]

Plasma AFP and eHCG levels are proportionally related to tumour volume. [42]
In the case of malignant seminomatous germ cell tumours, pure dysgerminomas have a non-secretory contingent. However, 5% of tumours contain syncytiotrophoblasts which produce ehCG. LDH and alkaline phosphatase are often non-specifically elevated. [44]
For non-seminomatous malignant germ cell tumours: yolk sac tumour with AFP secretion, choriocarcinoma with eHCG secretion and embryonal carcinoma and polyembryoma can both produce AFP and eHCG. [44]
Whereas embryonal carcinoma and immature teratomas may be pure or, in a third of cases, secret AFP (immature ovarian teratomas with foci of yolk sac tumour) [44].
Mixed germ cell tumours can also secrete eHCG, aFP, or both depending on the component.
Eighty-eight percent of ovarian germ cell tumours increased serum lactic dehydrogenase isoenzyme 1. [44] (tableXIII)

Table XIII: TGMO tumour markers.

Type de tumeur	AFP	HCG	LDH
Dysgerminome	-	+/-	+
Tumeur vitelline	+	+	+/-
Tératome immature	+/-	-	+/-
Carcinome embryonnaire	+/-	+/-	+/-
Choriocarcinome	-	+	+/-
Tumeur mixte	+/-	+/-	+/-

Apparently complete tumour exeresis must be accompanied by normalisation of markers within a maximum of 90 days.
An incomplete exercise should be suspected if rates stagnate or rise again. [42]
Although these markers are not specific, their measurement can provide prognostic information and may be useful in monitoring the disease to detect subclinical recurrence; for this reason, quantitative eHCG, aFP, lactic dehydrogenase and CA-125 should be measured preoperatively in all young women presenting with a pelvic mass. [45]
In our series, due to the rarity of germ cell tumours that were not initially considered, tumour marker assays were not performed pre-operatively in 73% of cases, and in most cases only a few markers (CA125, AFP) were assayed.

V. Anatomopathological study

1. Histological classification

Since 2003, the World Health Organisation has classified the different histological types of GIST into three main categories (Table XIV), and this classification includes all neoplasms derived histologically from the primordial germ cell epithelium of the embryonic gonad. [41]

Table XIV: Histological classification of TGMO.

Classification by the World Health Organization (WHO)	
Primary germ cell tumours	Dysgerminomas vitelline tumours (Volk sac tumors) Embryonal carcinoma Poly embryo me Non-gestational choriocarcinoma Mixed T
Biphasic or triphasic teratomas	Immature teratoma (grade according to glial component) Mature solid and cystic teratoma Tfiliform or homonculus
Monodermal teratoma	Struma ovarii group Grou p e c a rc i noTd e other malignant lesions

2. Anatomopathological examination

2.1. Dysgerminomas

On macroscopic examination, ovarian dysgerminomas are typically solid and well encapsulated, with an average diameter of 15 cm.

On sectioning, they are lobulated, fleshy and grey-white or light beige, with areas of necrosis and haemorrhage.

Dysgerminomas may be bilateral, with involvement of the contralateral ovary in 6.5% to 10% of cases [46-47].

The dysgerminomas in our series were straight in 85.7% of cases, bilateral in one case and purely solid in 71% of cases. They had a mean size of 16.5 cm.

The microscopic appearance of ovarian dysgerminomas is characteristic and identical to that of testicular seminomas. Ovarian dysgerminomas are composed of patches of uniform cells known as "seminomatous cells", divided into poorly demarcated lobules by fibrous strands and infiltrated by T lymphocytes. The cells have a clear eosinophilic cytoplasm and a large round or flattened central nucleus containing one or more prominent nucleoli. Mitoses are often numerous [41].

2.2. Yolk tumours

Yolk sac tumours are germ cell tumours whose cellular structure resembles that of the primitive yolk sac. The term yolk sac tumour is more inclusive than the term endodermal sinus tumour.

Yolk sac tumours present as large encapsulated masses with an average diameter of 15 cm and usually have a smooth external surface. In cross-section, they typically have mixed solid and cystic components. The solid components are grey to yellow, with extensive areas of hemorrhage and necrosis. Cysts vary from a few millimetres to 2 cm in diameter and are diffusely distributed throughout the tissue, giving the neoplasm an "alveolar appearance" [41].

Capsular tears, due to the rapid growth rate of these tumours, have been described on pathological examination and occur in 27% of cases [41]. Yolk sac tumours are bilateral in less than 5% of patients and the contralateral ovary contains a dermoid cyst in approximately 10% of cases [41].

In our series, the mean tumour diameter was 17cm, with a greyish-white colour and a smooth surface in both cases. They were solid cystic in 2/3 of cases.

Ten different histological profiles can be observed in yolk sac tumours: microcystic, sinus endodermal, solid, alveolar-glandular, polyvesicular vitelline, myxomatous, papillary, macrocystic, hepatoid and glandular. [46]

Schiller-Duval bodies are the most characteristic features of yolk sac tumours and correspond to papillary formations centred by a blood vessel in a cavity with a flattened epithelial lining. The presence of Schiller-Duval bodies may be considered diagnostic of a yolk sac tumour; however, in some cases they may be atypical or absent. Their absence does not exclude the diagnosis of yolk sac tumour if the tumour appearance is otherwise typical [46].

2.3. Non-gestational choriocarcinomas

The tumour is usually unilateral, between 4 and 25 cm in diameter, solid, greyish in colour and highly haemorrhagic. There is often a capsular rupture associated with hemoperitoneum. [48]

The typical appearance of choriocarcinoma is a plexiform arrangement of syncytiotrophoblast cells with mononuclear cells, mainly cytotrophoblasts, around foci of hemorrhage. [48]

Choriocarcinomas must be divided into gestational choriocarcinomas and non-gestational choriocarcinomas, which have immunohistochemical differences [48].

2.4. Embryonal carcinomas

In general, embryonal carcinomas are unilateral and large, with an average size of 17 cm. Macroscopically, they have a smooth outer surface and, on section, are soft, with a highly variable appearance and extensive areas of haemorrhage and necrosis. They are predominantly solid, with cystic spaces containing mucoid material. [49].

Embryonal carcinoma is characterised histologically by the presence of clusters of large pleomorphic cells that sometimes form papillae. The nuclei are usually large, crowded, pleomorphic and vesicular, with prominent nucleoli [50-51]. Embryonal carcinomas may occur in a pure form or as a component of a mixed germ cell tumour. The most common components associated with embryonal carcinomas in mixed germ cell tumours are yolk sac tumours and dysgerminomas [48].

The embryonal carcinomas in our series were solid in 80% of cases. They had an average size of 15 cm.

2.5. Polyembryomas

Polyembryomas are extremely rare TGMOs. Since their initial description, only 15 cases have been reported in the English medical literature, none of them in pure form but rather as a component of mixed GTTs in children and young women [46, 50, 51].

Immature teratomas and yolk sac tumours are the most frequently reported components associated with polyembryoma in mixed germ cell tumours. [51]

Polyembryomas are unilateral and large, with a microcystic surface. Microscopically, they consist of small embryoid-like bodies with central "germinal discs" composed of embryonal carcinoma epithelium and two cavities: a dorsal cavity resembling the amniotic cavity and a ventral cavity resembling the yolk sac cavity. The embryoid bodies are located in a redematous to myxoid stroma with prominent blood vessels [50].

2.6. Mixed germ cell tumours

Ovarian mixed germ cell tumours are composed of several germ cell elements, mainly dysgerminoma, teratoma and yolk sac tumour, although other elements such as choriocarcinoma, polyembryoma and embryonal carcinoma may be present [46].

In our series, the mixed germ cell tumour consisted of a grade II immature teratoma and an embryonal carcinoma.

2.7. Immature teratomas

Immature teratomas are usually unilateral. They contain immature or embryonic tissue, which distinguishes them from mature teratomas. [53] In general, immature teratomas are larger (14-25 cm) than mature cystic teratomas (mean 7 cm) [53]. Most immature teratomas are considered to be an encapsulated mass that is predominantly solid, soft and fleshy when cut. Small cysts may be present. Usually, cystic areas are filled with serous, mucinous or fatty sebaceous fluid. The cut surface is multinodular and brown to pink or grey to white. Frequently, areas of necrosis and haemorrhage are present. Fat, hair and sebaceous material may be seen [53].

In 26% of cases, a dermoid cyst is grossly identified in the immature cystic teratoma and in 10% of cases in the contralateral ovary [54].

The immature teratomas in our series had an average size of 17 cm; they were bilateral in one case, and most often solid-cystic (64.2%).

Microscopically, we see tissue derived from the three germ layers, with a variable mixture of mature and immature elements. The presence of immature elements establishes the diagnosis. The grading system for immature teratomas is based on the amount of immature neuroepithelium present. [53]

It has been clearly established that the amount of immature tissue has an indisputable prognostic significance. This parameter is the basis of histological prognostic grading, which most often uses the Scully and Thurlbeck system. [55] (Table XV)

Table XV: Histoprognostic grading of immature teratomas.

Grade	Thurlbeck and Scully
0	Good differentiation of all cell lines
	Well differentiated cells: rare small foci of embryonic tissue
2	Moderate amount of embryonic tissue: cellular atypia and mitoses present
3	Large quantity of embryonic tissue: cellular atypia and mitoses present

In our series, 14 immature teratomas were observed, representing 46.7% of cases, of which 57% were grade 1, 36% grade 2 and 7% grade 3.

3. Immunohistochemical profiles of TGMOs

Immunohistochemistry, a technique used in histology and cytopathology for over twenty years, has made considerable progress in cancer diagnosis and is widely used and useful in the positive and differential diagnosis of different histological subtypes of GIST.

A wide variety of markers are available, many of them new.

- **Dysgerminomas:** are generally immunoreactive for KIT in its membrane portion, CD2-40 in its cytoplasmic and membranous portion, and OCT-4 in its nuclear portion. Tumour cells are highly positive for stem cell markers such as SALL4 and are positive for PLAP, as are most malignant germ cell tumours. [43]

CD117 expression is present in >85% of all dysgerminomas. [43]

Some non-specific markers that are frequently positive are LDH, desmin, focal keratin positivity including CK7 can be found in a small proportion of cells.

Dysgerminomas are negative for EMA, ACE, CD30, glypican-3 (GPC3) and SOX2. Syncytiotrophoblastic cells are positive for HCG, GPC3, inhibin and keratins. [43]

In our series, CD117, PLAP and vimentin were positive, while dysgerminomas were negative for AFP, ACE, EMA and CD30.

- Unlike dysgerminomas**, yolk sac tumours** are immunoreactive for keratins**, GPC3** and **AFP** and negative for OCT4. The latter is the best marker for this differential diagnosis. KIT immunostaining is positive in a proportion of yolk sac tumours, particularly in solid areas, while D2-40 is negative. [43]

- Like dysgerminoma, embryonal carcinoma is positive for OCT4, but positivity for CD30 is found exclusively in embryonal carcinoma. In addition, embryonal carcinomas are differentially positive for keratins, whereas dysgerminomas are either negative or show only focal positivity. Most embryonal carcinomas are negative for KIT but about 30% are focally positive for D2-40. [43]

In our study, embryonal carcinomas were positive for CD30, EMA and keratin.

- **Choriocarcinomas**: all trophoblastic cells stain diffusely and strongly with keratins. CD 10 is positive in all trophoblastic cells in a membranous pattern. Approximately 50% of choriocarcinoma tumours are positive for PLAP and EMA. GPC3 is positive in most choriocarcinomas. Syncytiotrophoblastic cells stain positive for HCG and sometimes for human placental lactogen (HPL). SALL4 (nuclear) is positive in 70% of choriocarcinomas. [43]

- **Immature teratomas:** SALL4 positivity is observed in around 70% of immature neuroectodermal tissues of the immature ovary.

Immature neuroectodermal tissue in immature ovarian teratomas is positive for SOX2 and negative for NANOG. GPC3 can be positive in teratomatous glands and immature neuroepithelium and is therefore not useful in differentiating yolk sac tumour from mature or immature teratoma. [43]

In our study, teratomas were negative for AFP, EMA, keratin and CD30/CD20.

Table XVI: Immunohistochemical profiles of TGMO.

	SALL 4	OCT 4	CD 30	Keratin e	KIT	D2-40	AF P	SOX2	HCG
Dysgerminoma	**+**	**+**	**-**	**rare**	**+**	**+**	**-**	**-**	**Rare**
Yolk sac tumour	**+**	**-**	**-**	**+**	**certai n**	-	**+**	**-**	-

Embryonal carcinoma	**+**	**+**	**+**	**+**	**-**	**certain**	**-**	**certain**	**certain**
Choriocarcinomenon gestational	**+**	**-**	**-**	**+**	**-**	**-**	**-**	**-**	**+**
Immature teratoma	**+**	**+**	**-**	**-**	**-**	**-**	**-**	+	**-**

VI. Dissemination channels

Unlike epithelial ovarian cancer, in which intraperitoneal dissemination is the most common mode of spread and about 70% of patients have peritoneal metastases at diagnosis, lymphatic spread is the most common mode of spread for GIST [46-56].

Dysgerminomas spread late and are highly lymphophilic tumours. Tumour rupture may cause spillage of tumour contents and extensive peritoneal implantation. [46]

Yolk tumours are highly malignant and often invade surrounding structures, with extensive spread into the abdominal cavity. [56]

Yolk sac tumours and embryonal carcinomas metastasise early, mainly via the lymphatic system.

Immature teratomas spread by implantation throughout the peritoneal cavity and metastasise mainly through the lymphatic system. [57]

Choriocarcinomas are highly malignant and locally invasive, spreading widely throughout the abdominal cavity and metastasising early [57].

- **Local distribution**

Direct invasion into the pelvis most commonly involves the fallopian tubes, uterus and contralateral adnexa. With the exception of dysgerminomas, which are bilateral in 6.5% to 10% of patients, most BMTs are unilateral. [32-35] At a more advanced stage, the tumour extends to the bladder, rectum and pelvic walls.

- **Peritoneal dissemination**

Intra-peritoneal spread is a common pattern of spread in ovarian cancer, and BMT is no exception.

From the pelvis, normal peritoneal fluid flow carries tumour cells along the right paracolic gutter to the right upper quadrant, where implants are deposited on the hepatic capsule and diaphragmatic surface [56]. Tumour implants in the peritoneal cavity are most commonly seen in the cul de sac, paracolic gutters, epiploon, subphrenic space or mesentery.

Peritoneal metastases may be too small to be seen on imaging; when they are visible, they appear as thin nodular areas or sometimes thicker, giving the appearance of an epiploid cake. Mesenteric implants can distort and obstruct the bowel by causing adhesions or by frank invasion [56].

- **Lymphatic propagation**

The prevalence of lymph node metastases for all GCT subtypes is 18%. Dysgerminomas have the highest tendency for lymph node involvement, which is present in 28% of dysgerminomas, followed by mixed germ cell tumours, with metastatic adenopathy present in 16% of immature teratomas [3].

- **Distant metastases**

Hematogenous metastases are rare at the time of initial presentation; however, they may be seen in the liver and lungs in patients with recurrent disease.

Metastases to the brain, bone, suprarenal and other abdominal organs are much less common [56].

Stage IV disease is characterised by distant metastases. The most frequent finding of distant metastases in patients with GIST is malignant pleural effusion [56].

Hepatic parenchymal disease (stage IV) must be distinguished from capsular metastases (stage III).

VII. Anatomical and clinical classifications

The most commonly used stage classification is that of the FIGO international federation of obstetrics and gynaecology (table XVIIXVIII). [58]

This classification incorporates the most common modes of tumour spread, including direct invasion of pelvic structures and extension beyond the pelvis by intra-peritoneal, lymphatic or hematogenic diffusion.

Table XVII: FIGO 2018 classifications of epithelial tumours of the ovary. The early stages: IA-->IIA

Stages	Early
IA	Cancer confined to an ovary or tube. No tumour cells on the surface of the ovary or tube, or in the peritome.
IB	Cancer limited to the two ovaries or the two fallopian tubes. No tumour cells on the surface of the ovaries or fallopian tubes, or in the peritoneum.
IC	Cancer limited to one or two ovaries (one or two fallopian tubes)
IC1	Surgical rupture
IC2	Preoperative rupture or tumour cells on the surface of the ovary or tube
IC3	Tumour cells in peritoneal lavage
IIA	Involvement of one or two ovaries (or fallopian tubes) associated with pelvic extension below the superior strait (uterus, fallopian tube, ovary).

Table XVIII: FIGO 2018 classifications of epithelial tumours of the ovary. The advanced stages: IIB >IVB

Stages	Advance and metastatic
IIB	Extension to other pelvic organs
III	Involvement of the abdomen or lymph nodes
IIIA	Microscopic lymph node or abdominal suspicion
IIIA1	Isolated lymph node involvement
IIIA2	Microscopic abdominal +/- lymph node involvement
IIIB	Abdominal involvement <2 cm +/-ganglionic

IIIC Abdominal involvement > 2 cm +/- lymph nodes

IVA Pleural effusion with positive cytology
IVB Parenchymal or extra-abdominal metastasis

In our series, the tumour was classified as stage I in 56.7% of cases, stage II in 6.7% and stage III in 36.7%. None of the tumours were metastatic.

The FIGO classification is better suited to adenocarcinomas than to TGMOs.

There are several other more specific classifications of TGMOs which are used mainly in paediatric settings, such as :

- WOLLNER's classification. [59] (Table XIX).
- Pre- and post-operative TNM SFOP classifications. [42]

Table XIX: WOLLNER classification.

STADE	EXTENT OF THE DISEASE
I*	Exclusive atieinia of one ovary
11*	Atieinia of one or both ovaries with or without atieinia of the lumbo-aortic lymph nodes, without pelvic and/or abdominal extension.
III	Pelvic and/or abdominal extension
[V	Extra-abdominal metastatic atieinia

*Peritoneal cytology negative

VII.Treatment

The essential aim of treatment with TGMO is to cure patients while preserving ovarian hormonal function and subsequent fertility, and minimising the toxicity of the treatments.

1. Place of surgery

Surgery plays an important role in the treatment of TGMO. The aim of surgery is threefold:

- Diagnostic (determination of the histological type of tumour)
- Staging: This enables an inventory of the lesion to be made and the stage of the disease to be established.
- Therapeutic: removal of the tumour.

Initially the surgical guidelines for the management of MGT were modelled on the management of malignant epithelial tumours of the ovary. [42] It consists of: complete exploration of the pelvis and the entire abdominal cavity, total hysterectomy, bilateral adnexectomy, infra-colic omentectomy, appendectomy, pelvic and lumbo-aortic lymph node dissection, peritoneal biopsies, and maximum tumour reduction with digestive resection if necessary.

Malignant germ cell tumours of the ovary have certain characteristics that distinguish them from malignant epithelial tumours of the ovary. They are fast-growing cancers that can reach large dimensions, occur in young women of childbearing age and are chemo-sensitive and sometimes radiosensitive.

The surgical procedure has gradually become less invasive, with the aim of preserving the possibility of subsequent pregnancies, even in advanced stages.

The surgical procedure therefore consists of at least: unilateral adnexectomy, complete exploration of the pelvis and the entire abdominal cavity, peritoneal lavage and/or removal of any ascites present when the abdomen is opened, systematic peritoneal biopsies (including of the epiploon) and removal of any suspicious elements (biopsy of the contralateral ovary if there is a suspicious lesion and biopsies of the retroperitoneal lymph nodes). [62]
In what follows, we report on the various proposals for current surgical techniques aimed at optimising surgery for OMTs, taking into account their specific characteristics:
- **Laparotomy:** essential for palpation of the peritoneum, lymph nodes and contralateral ovary, and for removal of the tumour. The midline incision remains the technique of choice compared with crelioscopy, which, although effective for abdominal and pelvic exploration, is of limited use for large tumours and lymph node exploration. In addition, there is a risk of abdominal or parietal dissemination of neoplastic cells. [42, 61]
- **Peritoneal cytology:** if the ascites fluid or peritoneal lavage is not examined cytologically, there is a risk that stage Ic tumours will be overlooked and patients will be under-treated. This examination is therefore essential. [60, 61]

In our series, the surgical approach was by laparotomy in 80% of cases and peritoneal cytology was performed in 93% of cases.
- **Exploration of the abdominal cavity:** meticulous exploration of the entire pelvic cavity with biopsy of any suspicious areas is essential.
- **Adnexectomy** is preferred due to the existence of tumour cells in the tube in 30% of cases [61].
- **Contralateral ovary:** most studies agree that it is unnecessary if the contralateral ovary is macroscopically healthy. On the other hand, in the case of dysgerminoma, there is a risk of contralateral occult disease. Some authors therefore suggest that a contralateral biopsy should be carried out in such cases, without this having any impact on survival. However, it may lead to infertility [62-63].
- **Bilateral adnexectomy** is indicated when gonadal dysgenesis is discovered pre-operatively or per-operatively.

In our series, biopsy of the contralateral ovary was performed in 23% of cases, mainly for advanced tumours. It was negative in all cases.

1.1. The role of conservative surgery

Because of their chemosensitivity, the limited toxicity of chemotherapies, the excellent prognosis of TGMO and their occurrence in young children and adults, the majority of authors currently agree on abandoning aggressive surgery first. [64-65-66-67]
Conservative treatment should be carried out for all BMT regardless of histological type and tumour stage. [68-69]
For some authors, conservative treatment remains the treatment of choice regardless of histological type and tumour stage, but it should only be carried out after ruling out the gonadal dysgenesis frequently associated with BMT by means of a karyotype,

hormone assay and guided pelvic ultrasound. [25]
In our series, surgery was conservative in 23 patients (76.7%) and radical in 7 (23.3%).

1.2. The role of complete surgical staging

Initial surgery has been regarded as a staging operation, which is important in determining the extent of disease, providing prognostic information and guiding post-operative management [70].
Complete surgical staging is generally defined as unilateral salpingo-oophorectomy, omentectomy, peritoneal biopsies, peritoneal lavage and lymph node sampling. Ertas et al. reported that eight patients in their cohort had not completed surgical staging after detailed surgical exploration by experienced gynaecological oncologists. They considered that these patients had early stage disease, and none of them developed recurrence [71]. Similarly, Weinberg et al. reported in their cohort that surgical staging was not performed in only seven of 40 patients; none of the seven patients had recurrence [4].
Therefore, visual inspection has been suggested as an alternative approach to complete surgical staging [72]. This proposed surgical approach includes unilateral adnexectomy; inspection and palpation of the contralateral ovary, epiploon, lymph nodes and peritoneal surfaces; with biopsy of any suspicious lesions and peritoneal lavage [73].
The question of whether to repeat surgery in the case of inadequate staging is controversial. The experience of Tangjitgamol et al. showed that repeat surgery in their five patients appeared to have only limited benefit as the operations showed negative results, small residual unstaged tumours or advanced cancer where further surgery was not possible, while all required adjuvant chemotherapy [74].
Therefore, some authors have proposed that in localized GIST, complete staging or reclassification after inadequate initial surgery, if negative, allows safe observational management. The price to pay for incomplete staging is the same as for positive staging: chemotherapy containing cisplatin [75].
In our series, 16.6% of patients had an omentectomy and 33.3% had stage peritoneal biopsies.
Three patients with immature teratomas were reviewed for staging surgery and surgical totalization: the first had cystectomy alone (stage IA), the second had unilateral adnexectomy with contralateral lumpectomy for a stage IB tumor, and the third had unilateral adnexectomy for a stage IC tumor.

1.3. Place of lymph node surgery

The question that also arises in the management of MOGCT is whether patients with MOGCT should undergo systematic pelvic and para-aortic lymphadenectomy at the time of initial surgery.
In general, retroperitoneal recurrence in GIST is not well documented and the role of routine lymphadenectomy is unknown.
BMT is extremely chemo-sensitive. Most under-treated patients who have had a

recurrence can be recovered by chemotherapy, with excellent survival regardless of the extent of initial surgical staging [26]. This has been used as evidence to avoid systemic lymphadenectomy.

In addition, the lymph nodes must be explored radiologically before the operation.

During the surgical work-up, systematic radical lymph node dissection is no longer indicated because it has no impact on survival, at the cost of high morbidity [4266].

However, pelvic, external iliac and lumbo-aortic lymph nodes should be palpated and sampled if malignancy is suspected, as studies have shown that lymph nodes described as macroscopically abnormal by the surgeon are histologically tumourous in 41% of cases. [61]

For dysgerminomas, lymph node dissection is not systematic, even in the case of suspicious lymph nodes, due to the very high chemosensitivity and radiosensitivity of this histological type.

In our series, a per-operative verification of the lymph node areas was performed in 6 cases (this was mentioned in the medical observations). Lymph node dissection was performed in 3 patients, 2 of whom had stage IIIC dysgerminomas and the other a mixed germ cell tumour. It was positive in 2 of them.

To date, the value of lymph node testing in GIST remains controversial.

1.4. Place of second look surgery

The literature on the indications for surgery after chemotherapy is still open to debate. The cases reported are fewer in number and more heterogeneous. Second-look surgery has been used extensively in the past, and now makes it possible to better define the indications.

According to the reference centre for rare malignant gynaecological tumours [1] **second-look surgery is not indicated:**

- **For dysgerminomas**, even if retroperitoneal masses persist, they often do not contain living tumour cells and may continue to regress after CT.
- **For endodermal sinus tumours and choriocarcinomas**, which have sufficiently reliable tumour markers (alpha-FP and beta-HCG respectively) for monitoring purposes.
- **For patients diagnosed at an early stage and whose initial surgery has been completed.**

However, this surgery is necessary:

- **When only biopsies were taken** during the initial surgery.
- **In the case of embryonal carcinomas or non-secretory mixed germ cell tumours**, it is essential to assess the lesions remaining after chemotherapy.
- In the case of **"growing teratoma" syndrome**: This syndrome is a rare entity, defined by the growth of tumour masses in the retroperitoneal or other sites, occurring during or after chemotherapy for TGMND. Three criteria define this syndrome:

1-Increase in the size of the tumour mass.

2-Normal tumour markers.

3-Histologically: The tumour mass contains only mature teratomas.

It is the consequence of the existence within the tumour of a mature teratomatous contingent that is resistant to chemotherapy and can reach a large volume, causing functional complications. [77]

Although benign, growing teratoma is locally progressive and requires repeated surgery if resection is not complete. [78] Surgery is therefore essential. [21, 42]

No cases of growing teratoma were observed in our series.

1.5. The role of cytoreductive surgery

There is no doubt that early-stage GISTs have an excellent prognosis with standard treatment, while advanced tumours remain a challenge.

The role and extent of fertility-preserving cytoreductive surgery in patients with advanced BMT remains controversial despite its routine use [35]. Numerous studies have shown that residual tumour after surgery has a significant influence on overall survival and is the most important adverse prognostic factor [71]. In this respect, two studies from the gynaecological oncology group have shown that patients with unresectable or incompletely resected GIST had a lower chance of complete remission after chemotherapy than patients with minimal residual disease [79-80].

In the light of these reports, and given the chemotherapy-sensitive nature of BMD, an adequate attempt at maximal cytoreduction without compromising fertility appears to be a reasonable surgical approach in the initial treatment of young patients with advanced BMD, and current data have shown that maximal cytoreduction is significantly associated with improved overall survival. [81]

2. Adjuvant treatment

2. 1 Chemotherapy

Significant progress has been made in the treatment of patients with GIST over the last 40 years. Given the rarity of TGMO, studies of this type are difficult, but their similarity to testicular cancer has enabled researchers to extrapolate new treatments.

The evolution of combination chemotherapy for patients with GVHD began in the 1960s with the introduction of the combination of actinomycin-D, 5-fluorouracil and cyclophosphamide (AFC). Although several reports have documented modest success with this regimen, its popularity was short-lived, giving way to other combinations [8283].

During the 1970s, the combination of vincristine, actinomycin-D and cyclophosphamide (ACC) was popularised and became the standard treatment. This regimen resulted in a significant improvement in outcome, particularly for patients with stage I GIST, but led to remissions in only 50% of patients with stage III disease [84].

The major breakthrough in improving outcomes for patients with GIST occurred once cisplatin was introduced.

Einhorn and Donohue reported promising results in 1977 with the combination of vinblastine, bleomycin and cisplatin (PVB) for testicular cancer [85]. Subsequently, several reports have documented excellent results with this regimen in patients with GVHD [86].

Once Williams et al. reported an equivalent efficacy associated with a superior therapeutic index for the combination of bleomycin, etoposide and cisplatin (BEP) compared with the PVB regimen for men with testicular cancer [87], BEP was rapidly integrated into the treatment of patients with GVHD [88-89].
And for more than two decades, BEP chemotherapy has been the standard regimen at all stages of the disease [32].
After several studies comparing the toxicity of different chemotherapy protocols and their efficacy, BEP was shown to be superior to other protocols. [32]
With the exception of those with stage I immature teratoma and stage Ia dysgerminoma, all patients will have adjuvant chemotherapy [32,90].
The BEP protocol describes four cycles, every three weeks, with Bleomycin: 30 mg (D1, 8, 15), Etoposide: 100 mg/m^2 /D (D1, 5) and Cisplatin: 20 mg/m^2 /D (D1, 5).
BEP chemotherapy has significantly improved survival rates: 100% in patients with early-stage GBMT and 75% in those with advanced GBMT [32].
A review of the literature shows that 2 to 4 cycles of BEP achieve these high rates of curability. The majority of authors agree that 3 cycles of BEP should be administered in the case of complete tumour resection and 4 cycles in the case of incomplete resection. [91]
Chemotherapy containing a double dose of Cisplatin (200 mg/m^2 /D) has not been shown to be more effective than conventional dose chemotherapy [92] and should not be recommended.
Some patients do not respond to BEP-type therapy and are chemo-resistant to platinum.
Treatment failures are classified into two groups: either platinum-resistant (progression or recurrence during or within 4-6 weeks) or partially platinum-sensitive (reappearance 6 to 12 months after the end of treatment). [90]
There are very few data on the treatment of resistant TGMO patients, and most information is extrapolated from testicular cancer reports. Approximately 50% to 60% of patients with recurrent, partially platinum-sensitive testicular cancer can be saved with VeIP (vinblastine, ifosfamide and cisplatin) or TIP (paclitaxel, ifosfamide and cisplatin) therapy, with or without high-dose chemotherapy combined with hematopoietic stem cell reinjection. [90]
High-dose treatment with carboplatin, etoposide with or without cyclophosphamide, ifosfamide and/or paclitaxel may be superior to standard-dose treatment in these patients. [93]
Platinum-refractory patients are not curable. The published approach to salvage therapy is to provide a course of standard-dose VeIP, and if the patient responds, a second course of high-dose etoposide and carboplatin. [93]

2. 1.1. Neoadjuvant chemotherapy

In patients with generalized or locally advanced disease, neoadjuvant chemotherapy (NACT) may be justified.
Few trials, and certainly no randomised trials, are available to answer the question of

the utility of neoadjuvant chemotherapy in these patients. However, Talukdar et al. evaluated the use of neoadjuvant chemotherapy, using four cycles of BEP followed by fertility-preserving surgery in 23 patients with bulky disease, compared with 43 patients who underwent primary surgery with FIGO stage III or IV disease during the same period. [7]

Following neoadjuvant chemotherapy, 21 patients showed a response to treatment with 16 achieving a complete response and five with a partial response. Eighteen of the 21 patients in the neoadjuvant chemotherapy group were subsequently able to undergo fertility-sparing surgery, and those with residual disease received two additional cycles of BEP. 21 of the 23 patients survived with a median disease-free survival of 211 months. [7]

Lu et al. also studied the role of neoadjuvant treatment in a group of 127 women with yolk sac tumours. After a median follow-up period of 46 months, there was no significant difference in the recurrence rate between the NACT group and the primary surgery group. [8]

For women with advanced, bulky disease or medical co-morbidities, early studies suggest that NACT has an important role to play. [8]

Thus, the present study suggests that neoadjuvant chemotherapy may be a reasonable option in patients with extensive intra-abdominal disease, where initial surgery is associated with an increased risk of surgical morbidity, or initial tumour status precludes fertility-sparing conservative surgery.

2.1.2 Side effects of chemotherapy

Each of the drugs used in chemotherapy has its own toxicity, which is added to that of the others in the case of poly-chemotherapy.

In general, the uncontrolled distribution of drugs in systemic chemotherapy leads to acute toxicity of a hematological (CAV), digestive (vinblastine CAV), renal (EP, BEP, PVB), pulmonary (bleomycin), allergic, cutaneous, infectious, cardiac, otological (EP) and neurological (CAV) nature. [94]

It may be delayed and manifested by the same signs as acute toxicity, or by leukaemia, lymphomas (CAV, PVB) and by disorders of ovarian function (in the case of conservative treatment) of the ovarian failure type, although this remains rare. [94].

In our series, 14 patients underwent adjuvant chemotherapy (46.6%), which contained platinum salts in 100% of cases.

Of the 24 patients treated with chemotherapy, 21 (87.5%) underwent BEP chemotherapy. The average number of courses was 3.

Second-line chemotherapy was indicated in 4 patients: 3 cases of metastatic recurrence and one case of continued progression.

Complications of chemotherapy treatment were observed in 4 patients (16.7%):

- Hematological toxicity in a patient with anemia and neutropenia.
- Bleomycin-induced pneumonitis in a patient.
- Renal failure in two patients.

2. 2. targeted therapy

The role of targeted therapies in the treatment of GTT remains to be demonstrated. Some molecules have already been tested in testicular tumours.

Targeted therapy alone or in combination with chemotherapy could be a therapeutic option, but this needs to be better evaluated by prospective studies. [95]

2.3. Radiotherapy

Despite the remarkable radiosensitivity of dysgerminomas, radiotherapy is rarely recommended nowadays, as chemotherapy is more effective, much less toxic and preserves ovarian function.

Furthermore, in view of recent developments in chemotherapy, it is recognised that chemotherapy is more effective than irradiation of large volumes of healthy tissue, and is less likely to compromise salvage therapy in the event of relapse. In addition, given that most patients die of their ovarian tumour, and that most patients are relatively young at the time of diagnosis, due allowance should also be made for the delayed cancerogenic effects of radiation.

To date, no randomised trial has attempted to codify radiotherapy, hence its imperfectly established place, and its gradual abandonment because of its harmful effects on fertility and the chemosensitivity of dysgerminomas. [42- 96]

Radiotherapy was performed in our series for a stage IIA dysgerminoma in a 10-year-old girl.

3. Indications

In 2019, the French-speaking observatory for rare gynaecological malignant tumours codified the surgery for TGMO and initiated recommendations for surgical practice as well as for complementary treatment. [1] These recommendations are summarised in the following diagrams (Figure 39).

Initial clinical diagnosis should include ultrasound, thoracoabdominopelvic CT, and tumour markers including AFP, BHCG, LDH, and Ca-125.

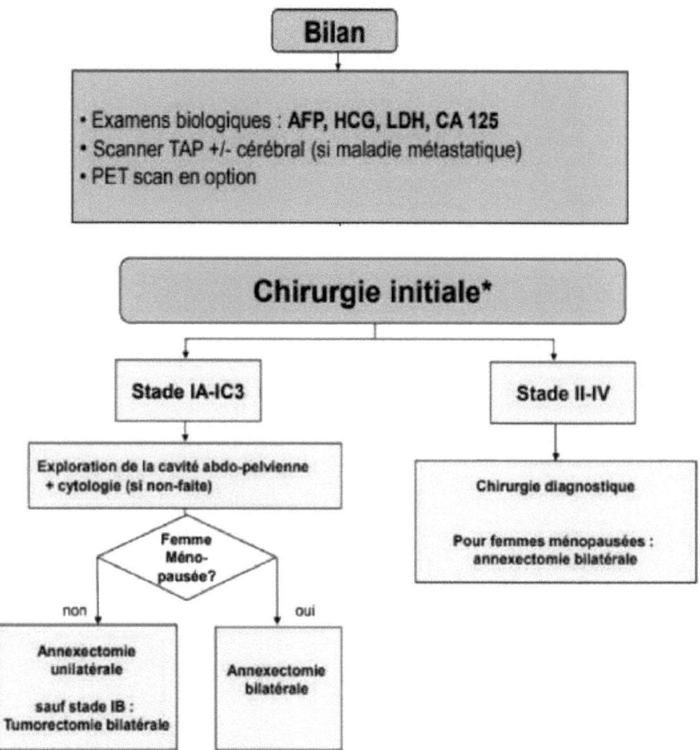

Figure 39: Initial management of TGMO [1].

The current recommendations for the complementary treatment of pure dysgerminoma, immature teratomas and vitelline tumours according to the Observatoire francophone des tumeurs malignes rares gynecologiques are summarised in the following diagram: (Figure 40- 41-42)

Additional treatment

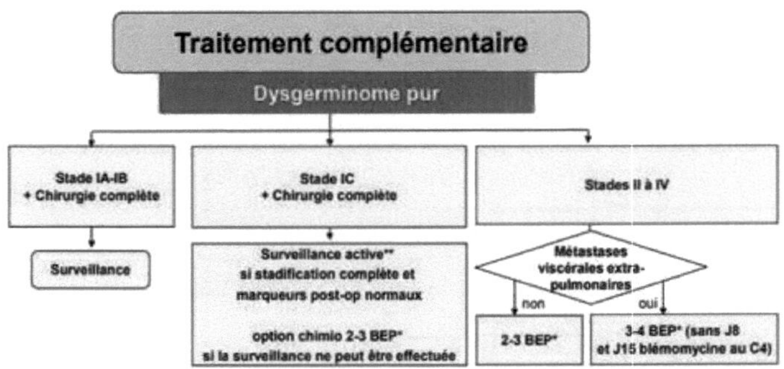

* **BEP** : cisPlatine 20 mg/m²/j J1 à J5 + Etoposide 100 mg/m² /j J1 à J5 + Bléomycine 30 mg J1, J8, J15 quelque soit la numération à J8 et J15
Surveillance de l'EFR pour les BEP seulement. Si altération de l'EFR, arrêt de la bléomycine
Discuter la réalisation de bléomycine chez les femmes > 40 ans.
Privilégier cisplatine etoposide (ou carboplatine-etoposide si cisplatine impossible) si > 60 ans

Pri vilegier cisplatin-etoposide (or carboplatin-etoposide if cisplatin impossible) if > 60 years old

Figure 40: Management of pure dysgerminomas according to FIGO stage

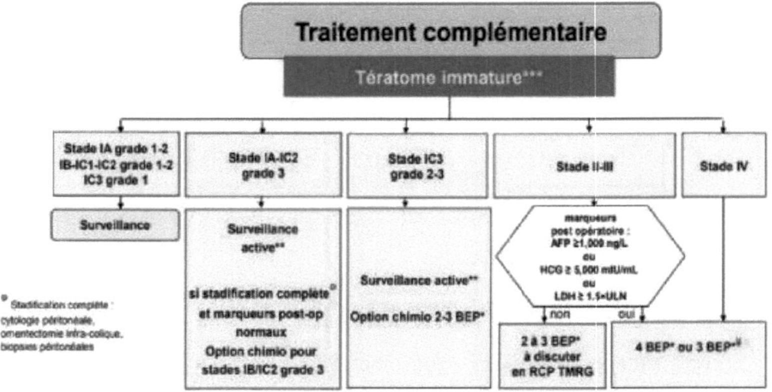

Figure 41: Management of immature teratomas according to stage and histological grade

¥ discuss 3 BEP if there are no extra-pulmonary visceral metastases and tumour markers are normal

*** Very close clinical and radiological monitoring during chemotherapy due to the risk of growing teratoma.

* BEP: cisPlatin 20 mg/m^2 /d D1 to D5 + Etoposide 100 mg/m^2 /d D1 to D5 + Bleomycin 30 mg D1, D8, D15 whatever the count at D8 and D15.

If EFR deteriorates, bleomycin should be stopped. Discuss the use of bleomyc:n in women over 40.

Additional treatment

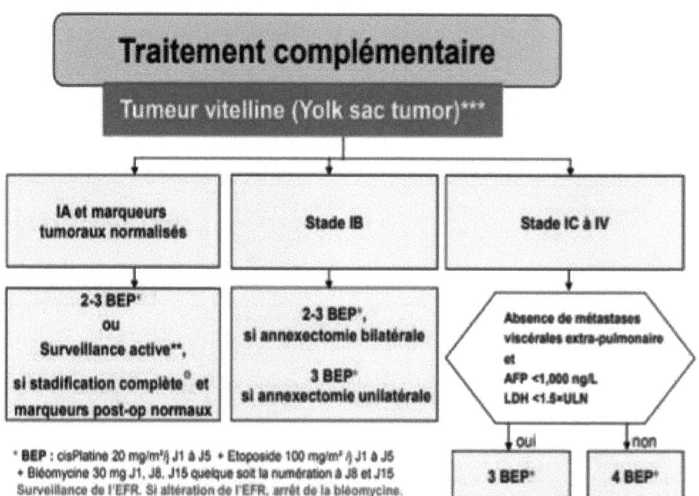

Complete staging: peritoneal cytology, infra-colic omentectomy, peritoneal biopsies

Figure 42: Management of yolk sac tumours according to FIGO stage

In order to standardise the language used by different therapists, the WHO (World Health Organisation) has classified the response to chemotherapy into 3 categories:

- A complete response: defined as the complete disappearance of all clinically detectable disease and the normalisation of tumour markers.
- A partial response was defined as a reduction of 50% or more in tumour size and a reduction in tumour markers.
- Progression is defined as an increase of more than 25% in the tumour compared with the best response or the appearance of new lesions. [7]

Based on these 3 types of response, the management of TGMO after chemotherapy according to the Observatoire francophone des tumeurs malignes rares is summarised in the following diagram:(Figure 43)

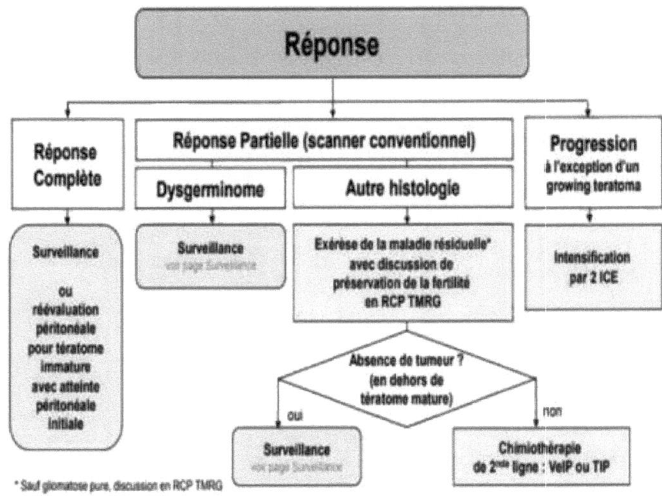

Figure 43: Complementary management according to therapeutic response

ICE: Etoposide 300 mg/m^2 /d 5 days (staggered infusion: 150 mg/m^2 every 12 hours for 5 days), ifosfamide 2.4 g/m^2 /d 5 days, Carboplatin AUC 4/day 5 days.
Total: etoposide 1500 mg/m2, carboplatin AUC 20, ifosfamide 12 g/m2
VeIP: Vinblastine + Ifosfamide + cisPlatinum
TIP: placliTaxel + Ifosfamide + Platinum

VIII.Evolution

1. Recurrence and metastases

1.1. Dysgerminomas

Although recurrence of dysgerminoma is rare, 75% will occur within the first year after initial treatment [97]. Only a few cases of recurrence occurring after the first two years have been reported in the literature. [98]

The contralateral ovary, pelvis and retroperitoneal lymph nodes are the sites most frequently affected by dysgerminoma extension. [97]

Distant metastases are rare; they occur via the hematogenic route and preferentially affect the liver (90% of cases), lung, bone and brain. [99]

In our study, metastatic progression was observed in a patient with stage IIIC dysgerminoma, for whom surgery was incomplete. Metastases developed in the liver after 4 months of surgical treatment. The patient died six months later.

1.2. NDT

Unlike dysgerminomas, 90% of non-dysgerminomatous malignant germ cell tumours recur within the first two years. NMDGTs have a poor prognosis when they relapse, with a long-term survival rate of 10%. [97]

Embryonal carcinoma and yolk sac tumour are the most aggressive tumours among the TGMOs. They metastasise rapidly by both lymphatic and hematogenic routes and invade neighbouring organs and the entire peritoneal cavity. [96]

Immature teratomas are characterised by a rapid increase in size. Recurrence occurs fairly rapidly, especially if the tumour mass has ruptured spontaneously or during surgery. [102] Dissemination occurs via the peritoneal route, giving gliomatosis peritoneum, via the lymphatic route involving the iliac and lumbo-aortic lymph nodes, and via the blood to the liver and lungs. [101]. Recurrence is much more frequent in cases of grade 3 and 2 immature teratoma. [101]

The long-term prognosis of non-gestational choriocarcinoma is difficult to establish because of its rarity.

The evolution of mixed germ cell tumours is similar to that of their histological types. [96]

The current recommendations for chemotherapy of GTT in the event of recurrence or progression of the disease according to the Francophone observatory of rare gynaecological malignancies are summarised in the following diagram: (Figure 44)

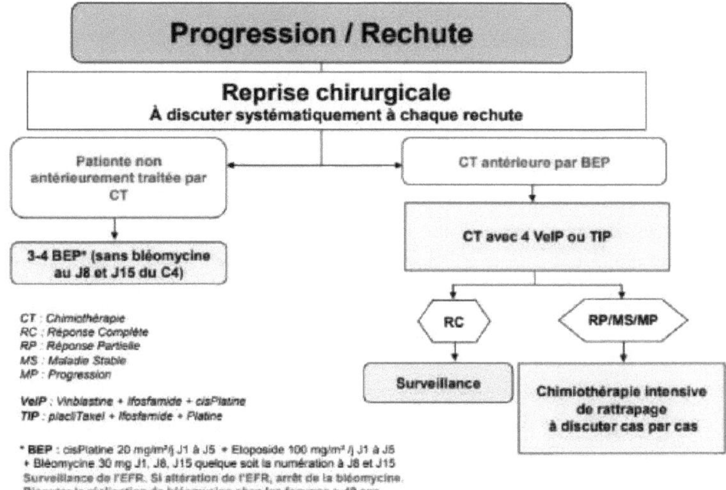

Figure 44: Therapeutic management of tumour progression or relapse

We observed 2 metastatic recurrences occurring 24 and 48 months after diagnosis in two patients with immature teratomas classified as stage IA and IIIA, after initial conservative surgical treatment in both cases, but these patients did not respond to chemotherapy. Both patients developed supraclavicular and mediastinal lymph node metastases.

The third metastatic recurrence occurred in a patient who had undergone chemotherapy followed by radical treatment for a stage IIIB mixed germ cell tumour. Pelvic and lumbo-aortic curage was positive in this patient and surgery was complete. The patient was in complete remission after 120 months. In this patient, the metastases were located in the pleuropulmonary region and in the supra-clavicular lymph nodes.

All three patients underwent 2[eme] lines of chemotherapy.

2. Fertility

Fertility is a key issue, given the young, even very young, age of diagnosis in patients who are generally nulliparous and have a disease with an excellent overall prognosis.

All authors currently agree on the need for treatment to preserve fertility in young patients with GIST.

This fertility can be preserved in patients treated by conservative surgery with or without chemotherapy.

Platinum-based chemotherapy, in particular the BEP regimen, respects patients' ovulatory function and preserves their hopes of fertility. [103]

Recent studies of reproductive function after fertility surgery followed by chemotherapy for OMT have shown that 80% to 99% of patients return to a normal menstrual cycle within six months of treatment [104].

Overall, the results on ovarian hormonal function and fertility in patients treated with conservative surgery and chemotherapy are good. In recent studies of TGOM, approximately 75% of women were able to conceive a child [105-106]. The rate of infertility reported in women trying to conceive after treatment for TGOM varies from 5% to 10%. [107]. This rate is similar to the rate of infertility in the normal population. [104]

There does not appear to be an excess of miscarriages compared with the general population. In fact, in an examination of 169 women by Zanetta et al, a miscarriage rate of 11% was recorded, which does not differ from the general population. On the other hand, no statistical difference was found in the rates of congenital malformation between women who received chemotherapy and those who did not. [108]

The association of TGMO and pregnancy is rare, representing only 2 to 5% of all malignant ovarian tumours diagnosed during pregnancy. [37]

Given the absence of hormone dependence in this type of tumour, and the probable absence of a link between BMT and hormone replacement therapy (HRT), HRT may be used in a woman previously treated for BMT.

Similarly, given the absence of a probable link between TGMO and hormonal contraception, all contraceptive methods can be used in these patients. [109]

In our series, we did not study the average recovery time for normal menstrual cycles.

Among ten women attempting pregnancy, nine were able to conceive, including two with stage III at the time of diagnosis, further confirming that conservative treatment should be recommended even at advanced stages.

The data from our study confirm that normal gonadal function and fertility are possible after conservative surgery for malignant ovarian germ cell tumours, even in the presence of chemotherapy.

No association between TGMO and pregnancy was observed in our series.

IX. Prognostic factors and survival

1. Survival

The different overall survival rates reported in the literature demonstrate the good prognosis of these tumours and their relatively good response to treatment.

According to the American Cancer Society (ACS), 5-year overall survival rates for the different types of GIST range from 69% for FIGO stage IV to 98% for FIGO stage I. [110] (Table XX)

Table XX: Five-year survival rate for TGMO according to FIGO stage.

FIGO Stadium	ACS survival rate	Our results
I	98%	94.7%
II	94%	100%
III	87%	73.2%
IV	69%	-

The overall and 5-year survival of TGMOs varies considerably according to subtype.

- Dysgerminomas have a very favourable prognosis. In the early stages, they have a 5-year survival rate of 96.9%. [96] **In our series, this was 100%.**

Stage III dysgerminomas have a five-year survival of 61%; and for dysgerminomas treated with BEP chemotherapy after incomplete surgical resection have a two-year survival rate of 95%[96].

- For pure immature teratomas, the 5-year survival rate for all stages combined is 70-80%, and 90-95% for stage I [97].

In our series, VT and MGT were the histological types associated with the lowest survival rates. This is consistent with data from the MITO9 study [5].

Table 20 shows a comparison of survival rates according to histological type in our study and that of MITO9.

Table XXI: Comparison of OS at 5 years between our study and the MITO9 study.

Histological type	SG is 5 years old in the study MITO9 (%)	SG at 5 years in our study (%)
Dysgerminoma	100	85.7
Immature teratoma	97.9	85.7
Yolk tumour (VT)	69.6	66.7
Mixed germ cell tumour (MGCT)	68.7	0%

2. Prognostic factors

Several series have attempted to identify prognostic factors capable of establishing metastatic risk.

In our series, the search for possible factors predictive of survival is complicated by the low number of events (death or recurrence) observed during the patient follow-up period.

The known poor prognostic factors in TGMO are :

- **Age:** Opinions are divided according to the authors. Indeed, for some, this factor does not constitute a fundamental prognostic element, whereas others support the idea that an age greater than 22 years is an interesting prognostic factor [111].

In our series, age over 30 years was a poor prognostic factor.

- **There is an advanced stage at the time of diagnosis**: stages III and IV [32]; all authors agree that survival is better in the early stages.

Our results are consistent with those reported in the literature, in that the 5- and 10-year survival of patients classified as stage I and II was better than that of patients classified as stage III. Indeed, the 5- and 10-year OS of patients classified as stage I and II was 94.7%, and that of patients classified as stage III was 73.2%.

- **Histological type and high histological grade** (for immature teratomas) [32] All authors agree that dysgerminomas have a better prognosis, whereas vitelline tumours and choriocarcinomas are the most aggressive TGMNDs.

Given the higher incidence of immature teratomas in our series, the OS of patients with dysgerminomas was comparable to that of patients with immature teratomas.

Similarly, the prognosis for immature teratomas is related to both stage and grade. In the study by Jorge et al (1045 cases of TI), the 5-year OS of grade I immature teratomas was better than that of grade II and grade III immature teratomas. [112]. Histological grade was not a prognostic factor in our study.

- **Initial marker levels:** The prognostic value of high AFP levels remains controversial. In paediatric studies, a better prognosis has been found when the initial AFP level is greater than 10,000 ng/ml [113]. However, studies that have specifically evaluated the prognostic value of this marker in patients with vitelline tumours have not found a significant correlation between preoperative AFP level and prognosis [57-114-115].

In our study, tumour marker assays were carried out in only 60% of patients, and were incomplete in most cases.

- A tumour residue greater than 1 cm after surgery following chemotherapy is a decisive prognostic factor [96].

Here too, the majority of authors agree that the most complete tumour excision possible improves survival. [116-117-118]

Only one case of incomplete surgery after neoadjuvant chemotherapy was noted in our series; it was a stage IIIC dysgerminoma and the evolution was marked by tumour progression with death after 12 months.

- The absence of platinum salts in the initial chemotherapy, insufficient doses or inadequate duration [41].
- Patients who are refractory to platinum salts [119] or who relapse very rapidly after a full course of chemotherapy also have a poor prognosis [118].
- **Tumour rupture** is thought to reduce the 5-year survival rate by 30% [120].
- **Lymph node status:** The value of lymph node dissection in TGMO remains controversial.

Kumar et al. reported that lymph node involvement is an independent prognostic factor. Indeed, the 5-year OS in the absence of lymph node involvement was better than in the presence of lymph node involvement (95.7% versus 82.8%, $p<0.001$). [121]

However, other studies had different results. Mahdi et al. analysed 493 MOGCT who underwent lymphadenectomy versus 590 patients who did not undergo this procedure and found that neither lymphadenectomy nor lymph node metastasis was an independent prognostic factor for survival [122]. Others have found that performing systemic lymphadenectomy in early stage patients can only define stages, but cannot significantly improve prognosis [123].

Our results could neither affirm nor confirm these studies, as only three patients had undergone lymph node dissection.

- **Tumour size greater than 10 cm** [38]: Opinions are divided according to the authors. For some, this factor is not a fundamental prognostic factor, while others support the opposite hypothesis.

In our series, a tumour size greater than 20 cm was a poor prognostic factor. In fact, for tumours >20 cm in size, survival at 5 and 10 years was 60%, and for those <20 cm in size, it was 100% at 5 years (P = 0.004).

- **Type of surgery:** The vast majority of authors agree that radical surgery does not improve the prognosis of GIST.

In the studies by Zanetta et al. and Chan et al. the fact that the surgical treatment was conservative did not seem to affect the prognosis [108-124]. Similarly, in the MITO9 study, there was no significant difference in terms of recurrence rate between patients who had undergone conservative surgery (17.4%) and those who had undergone radical surgery (19.3%). [5]

In our series, there was no significant difference between radical and conservative treatment in terms of overall survival.

Other poor prognostic factors have been reported in the literature, such as

- a low educational and socio-economic level, [125]
- **Marital status**: in fact, the best results were observed in married women, and this may be explained by better adherence to treatment and better access to care. [126]
- **Pregnancy** has no direct influence on prognosis, but it does delay the onset of the disease.

both the diagnosis and the initiation of treatment. [127]

X. Surveillance

Only rigorous and prolonged post-operative monitoring will enable recurrences to be diagnosed early and treatment resumed.

This monitoring is based on physical examination, biology (particularly for secreting tumours) and radiology.

Stage Ic dysgerminoma, immature teratomas with poor prognosis factors (grade 3, IC3) and stage IA vitelline tumours not treated with adjuvant chemotherapy should be actively monitored at more frequent intervals.

According to the Observatoire francophone des tumeurs malignes rares gynecologiques (French-speaking observatory of rare gynaecological malignant tumours), the surveillance methods for TGMO are summarised in Figure 45 :

Active Surveillance					
Monitoring	1'* annëe	2ëте annëe	3rd anëe	4ëте annëe	5ëй1Оё annëe
Clinical examination	/ month	/ 2 months	/ 3 months	/ 4 months	/ 6 months
Biology (AFP HCG. LDH GA 125 seton secretxxi mcrafe)	/ 15 days, for the first 6 months) then / month	/ 2 months	13 months	1 4 months	/ 6 months
TAP scanner	the 1*" month unontM the 3*™ month s> o "n stao" the i2tr ™! months				
Pelvic ultrasound	/ 2 words	/4 months	/ 6 months		
Chest X-ray	/ 2 months	/ 4 words	/ 6 months	/ 8 months	/ year
PET-scan for pure dysgerminoma	1" month к no "M then / 3-6 months	A rexuncucn d" r6itou*			

Surveillance end of tra items nt			
Monitoring	1"-2*"* annëe	3*'n *-5*"'* annëe э	5*"* annëe
Technical examination	7 3-6 months	t 6 months	i year
Biology [AFP. нес, LDH, CA 125setan заегёиэт mibdek	/ month for the first 3 months then t 3 months		/ в month f year
EFR completes, el clairance creatinine, si anormaies	End of chemotherapy and 126 words		
TAP scan ($i stage > 1)	13-6 months	i	anfan
Pelvic ultrasound for conservative treatment	! 3-6 months	/ 5 months	fan
PET-scan for pure dysgerminoma	1 e 1month if not ім pLJiiS / 3-6 months JuequA Гвмтсъ&п dei te-udui		

Figure 45: surveillance methods for TGMO according to the 1 observatoire francophone des tumeurs malignes rares gynecologiques.

BEP chemotherapy is the regimen of choice in advanced MOGCT, while there is now a trend towards narrow surveillance in stage 1 surgical MOGCT.

After fertility-preserving surgery and BEP chemotherapy, most women will return to their original menstrual function.

Fertility rates are close to those of the normal population, with no significant increase in the risk of early pregnancy loss or teratogenicity.

5 CONCLUSION

Malignant germ cell tumours of the ovary are rapidly growing tumours that derive from germ cells.

of the ovary. They represent around 2% to 3% of all ovarian cancers in Western countries and 29% of all malignant germ cell tumours. They are heterogeneous and are classically subdivided into dysgerminomatous tumours and non-dysgerminomatous tumours.

They generally occur in the first two decades of life, with an incidence rate of 75% in women under 30 and a peak between the ages of 15 and 25.

These tumours therefore pose a problem in terms of management, which must meet the carcinological imperatives while trying to preserve fertility.

Our work is a retrospective study of 30 cases of malignant germ cell tumours of the ovary diagnosed in the Gynecology-Obstetrics, Medical Oncology and Anatomopathology Departments of the FARHAT HACHED University Hospital in Sousse over a period of 21 years (1st September 1998 to 30th September 2019).

The average age of our patients was 22, with extremes ranging from 10 to 40.

The age of onset varies according to the histological type: 17 years for dysgerminoma, 35 years for yolk sac tumour and 25 years for immature teratoma.

The majority of patients (93.3%) were genitally active, two-thirds of whom were nulliparous.

The average consultation time was less than 6 months in 70% of cases.

The circumstances of discovery were varicose veins, dominated by abdomino-pelvic pain in 24 patients, and increased abdominal volume in 5 cases. Tumour torsion with an acute abdomen was the circumstance in one case. In one of our patients, the discovery was fortuitous following a thromboembolic accident.

Tumour marker assays were carried out in only 22 patients, and were often incomplete.

AFP was measured in 22 patients; it was pathological in 15.

The HCG assay was pathological in 2 out of 6 patients, and the LDH assay was carried out in only 4 patients, and was pathological in one case.

Abdominopelvic ultrasound was performed in 80% of our patients, showing a suspicious appearance of malignancy in 100%. The most characteristic appearance was a heterogeneous parenchymal echogenic mass with sharp margins and high vascularity.

The tumours were bilateral in 13% of cases, on the left ovary in 28% and on the right ovary in 50% of patients; the average size was 14 cm.

Ultrasound revealed ascites in 9 patients, with small amounts in 73% of cases.

Computed tomography (CT) and magnetic resonance imaging (MRI) were performed to investigate the etiology of a large pelvic mass of undetermined origin or as part of an extension assessment. CT was performed in 11 patients, 100% of whom had tumours larger than 150 mm. It confirmed the ultrasound findings and showed tumours of heterogeneous appearance in 10 cases. In addition, the CAT scan did not show any

secondary sites or lymph node involvement in all cases.
The management of TGMO depends on the stage of extension of the tumour, the desire for pregnancy and the histological type.
In our study, stage I was predominant in 17 patients (56.7%), stage II in 2 (6.7%), stage III in 11 (36.7%) and stage IV in none.
There were 7 cases of dysgerminomas, 14 cases of immature teratomas, 3 cases of vitelline tumours, 5 cases of embryonal carcinomas and 1 case of mixed tumours.
Surgery plays a major role in the management of malignant germ cell tumours of the ovary. It enables the diagnosis to be made, the stage of the disease to be determined and, in the majority of cases, the first therapeutic procedure to be carried out.
Conservative treatment should be offered whenever possible, due to the chemosensitivity of these tumours, their good prognosis and the fact that they occur in young patients who wish to become pregnant.
Fertility-sparing surgery with surgical staging is therefore the standard surgical approach for these ovarian tumours.
The current consensus is that as complete a tumour excision as possible improves survival, while the role of aggressive radical surgery in these chemosensitive tumour types is not well defined.
For our patients, 21 (70%) were approached by midline laparotomy, given the volume of the tumour, and only 9 by crelioscopy.
In terms of type of surgery, 23 patients (76.7%) underwent conservative treatment, leaving the ovary and uterus in place.
Peritoneal cytology was the first procedure performed in 93.3% of cases.
Ovarian biopsy and peritoneal biopsy were the procedures performed for stage III tumours in 63.3% and 90.9% of cases respectively.
Nowadays, the value of lymph node dissection remains controversial. Extensive and systematic lymph node curage is not currently recommended, and lymph node procedures should be limited to sampling suspected lymph nodes if necessary (after palpation and verification of all lymph node territories during surgery).
Lymph node surgery was performed in 10% of our patients (3 patients).
The literature on the indications for second-look surgery is still open to debate and its value is controversial.
The prognosis of BMT has been considerably improved by the introduction of adjuvant cisplatin-based chemotherapy. BEP-type chemotherapy is now the treatment of choice for GIST.
The BEP protocol was used in 85.7% of cases. Adjuvant chemotherapy was administered to 14 of our patients (46.6%) and neoadjuvant to 10 (33.3%). The mean number of courses was 3.5.
Radiotherapy has almost been abandoned nowadays because of its side effects. It was performed on a single 10-year-old patient with a stage IIA dysgerminoma.
Rigorous surveillance is essential after treatment for malignant germ cell tumours of the ovary, as the majority recur within the first two years (15-25% for

dysgerminomas).

In our series, patients were followed for an average of 94 months.

We observed one patient with incomplete resection of a stage IIIC dysgerminoma and 3 cases of metastatic recurrence which occurred after a mean period of 48 months, with extremes ranging from 24 to 120 months.

The two cases of recurrence were observed in patients who had not received adjuvant treatment: one was an immature teratoma stage IA grade III and the second was stage IIIA. The third recurrence was a stage IIIB mixed germ cell tumour that had undergone radical surgery with positive pelvic and lumbo-aortic curage.

Metastases occurred in the liver, lung, mediastinum and supra-clavicular lymph nodes.

Salvage treatment consisted of second-line chemotherapy in all cases.

The overall survival of GISTs reported in the literature demonstrates the good prognosis of these tumours and their relatively good response to treatment. This 5-year survival, all types combined, varies from 69% to 98% according to the American Cancer Society.

Overall survival at 5 and 10 years in our series was 85.7% and 75.8% respectively.

The prognostic factors for the isolated malignant germ cell tumours of the ovary in our series were consultation time greater than 6 months, age greater than 30 years, tumour size greater than 20 cm and tumour stage.

Following fertility-preserving surgery and BEP chemotherapy, most women will return to their initial menstrual function. Fertility rates thus approach those of the normal population, without any significant increase in the risk of early pregnancy loss or teratogenicity.

In our study, out of 106 women attempting pregnancy, 9 were able to conceive, including 2 who were stage III at the time of diagnosis, thus confirming that conservative treatment should be recommended even at advanced stages.

The data from our study also confirm that normal gonadal function and fertility are possible after conservative surgery for malignant ovarian germ cell tumours, even in the presence of chemotherapy.

In conclusion, the main findings from comparing our results with those in the literature are as follows:

- On imaging, dysgerminoma, the most common malignant germ cell tumour, usually appears as a solid mass.

Immature teratomas appear as a solid mass with scattered foci of fat and calcifications.

Yolk sac tumours usually present as a mixed solid and cystic mass. Capsular rupture or bright spot sign, resulting from increased vascularisation and formation of small vascular aneurysms, may be present.

Embryonal carcinomas and polyembryomas rarely occur in a pure form and are usually part of a mixed germ cell tumour.

- Tumour markers are useful for diagnosis and post-treatment follow-up. They should be measured systematically before surgery.
- Surgery plays a major role in the management of malignant germ cell tumours of

the ovary. It enables the diagnosis to be made, the exact stage of the tumour to be determined and, in the majority of cases, the first therapeutic procedure to be carried out.

- Conservative treatment should be offered whenever possible, because of the chemosensitivity of these tumours, their good prognosis and the fact that they occur in young patients who wish to become pregnant.
- BEP-type chemotherapy is the unanimous choice of the authors.
- Second-look surgery is still under discussion.
- Systematic lymph node dissection is not currently recommended.
- Radiotherapy has almost been abandoned nowadays.
- Rigorous post-therapy monitoring is essential.

6 REFERENCES

[1] Expert centre for rare gynaecological malignancies - May 2019 version.

[2] Brown J, Friedlander M, Backes FJ, et al. Gynecologic Cancer Intergroup (GCIG):consensus review for ovarian germ cell tumors. Int J Gynecol Cancer. 2014;24:S48-54.

[3] Kumar S, Shah JP, Bryant CS, et al. The prevalence and prognostic impact of lymph node metastasis in malignant germ cell tumors of the ovary. Gynecol Oncol. 2008;110:125-32.

[4] Weinberg LE, Lurain JR, Singh DK, Schink JC. Survival and reproductive outcomes in women treated for malignant ovarian germ cell tumors. Gynecol Oncol. 2011;121:285-9.

[5] Mangili G, Sigismondi C, Gadducci A, Cormio G, Scollo P et al. Outcome and risk factors for recurrence in malignant ovarian germ cell tumors: a MITO-9 retrospective study. Int J Gynecol Cancer. 2011;21:1414-21.

[6] Gershenson DM, Frazier AL. Conundrums in the management of malignant ovarian germ cell tumors: Toward lessening acute morbidity and late effects of treatment. Gynecol Oncol. 2016;143:428-32.

[7] Talukdar S, Kumar S, BhatlaN, Mathur S, Thulkar S, Kumar L. Neoadjuvant chemotherapy in the treatment of advanced malignant germ cell tumors of ovary. Gynecol Oncol. 2014;132:28-32.

[8] Lu Y, Yang J, Cao D, Huang H, Wu M, You Y. Role of neoadjuvant chemotherapy in the management of advanced ovarian yolk sac tumor. Gynecol Oncol. 2014;134:78-83.

[9] Yu HH, Yonemura Y, Hsieh MC, Lu CY, Wu SY, Shan YS. Experience of applying cytoreductive surgery and hyperthermic intraperitoneal chemotherapy for ovarian teratoma with malignant transformation and peritoneal dissemination. Therapeutics and Clinical Risk Management. 2019;15: 129-136.

[10] Kaatsch P, Hafner C, Calaminus G, Blettner M, Tulla M. Pediatric germ cell tumors from 1987 to 2011: incidence rates, time trends, and survival. Pediatrics. 2015; 135 (1):136-43.

[11] Matz M, Coleman MP, Sant M, Chirlaque MD, Visser O, Gore M, Allemani C. The histology of ovarian cancer: worldwide distribution and implications for international survival comparisons (CONCORD-2). Gynecologic Oncology. 2017;144 (2): 405-413.

[12] Hinchcliff .E, Diver.E, Hall.T, Stall.J et al, Racial disparities in survival in malignant germ cell tumors of the ovary, Gynecol Oncol. 2016; 140: 463-9.

[13] Oberaigner W, Minicozzi P, Bielska-Lasota M, Allemani C, de Angelis R, Mangone L et al. Eurocare Working Group. Survival for ovarian cancer in Europe: The across-country variation did not shrink in the past decade. Acta Oncol. 2012; 51:441-53.

[14] Smith HO, Berwick M, Verschraegen CF et al. Incidence and survival rates for female malignant germ cell tumors. Obstet Gynecol. 2006;107:1075-1085.

[15] Gershenson Dm, Del Junco G, Copeland Lj, Rutledge Fn. Mixed germ cell tumors of the ovary. Obstet Gynecol 1984; 64:200-6.

[16] Brookfield KF, Cheung MC, Koniaris LG, Sola JE, Fischer AC. A population-based analysis of 1037 malignant ovarian tumors in the pediatric population. J Surg Res. 2009;156:45-49.

[17] Quirk JT, Natarajan N, Mettlin CJ. Age-specific ovarian cancer incidence rate patterns in the United States. Gynecol Oncol. 2005;99:248-250.

[18] M0ller H, Evans H. Epidemiology of gonadal germ cell cancer in males and females. APMIS. 2003;111:43-48.

[19] Guillem V, Poveda A. Germ cell tumours of the ovary. Clin Transl Oncol. 2007;9:237-243.

[20] Chien O, Ady K, Enrique H. Ovarian Endodermal Sinus Tumor in a Postmenopausal Woman. Gynecol Oncol . 2001; 82: 392-4.

[21] Ray-Coquard I, Gustalla IP, Treilleux I, Biron P, Blay J-Y, Curie H. Malignant ovarian tumors. Oncology. 2005; 7 : 556-563.

[22] Tian Q, Fierson Hf, Krystal Gw, Moshaluk Ca. Activating Kit gene mutations in human germ cell tumors. Am J Path. 1999; 154:1643-7.

[23] Kraggerud SM, Hoei-Hansen CE, Alagaratnam S, Skotheim RI, Abeler VM et al. Molecular characteristics of malignant ovarian germ cell tumors and comparison with testicular counterparts: implications for pathogenesis. Endocrine Reviews. 2013;34 (3): 339-76.

[24] Cyriac S, Rajendranath R, Robert LA, Sagar TG. Familial germ cell tumor. Indian J Hum Genet. 2012;18:119-121.

[25] Rzepka-Gorska I, Blogowska A, Zajaczek S, Zielinska D. Germinal cell tumors in young and adolescent girls. Ginekol Pol. 2003; 9:840-6.

[26] Ben Romdhane K, Bessrour A, Ben Amor Ms, Ben Ayed M. Pure gonadal dysgenesis with gonadoblastoma, dysgerminoma and embryonal carcinoma. Bull Cancer 1988; 75:263- 9.

[27] Caponetti R, Caponetti D, Delogu D. Multiple ovarian cancer histotypes in a patient affected by Swyer syndrome. Gynecol Oncol. 2006;102:411-4. [28] Germa Jr, Iziquierdo Ma. Malignant ovarian germ cell tumors: the experience at the hospital de la Santa Creu I Sant Pau. Gynecol Oncol 1992; 45: 153-9.

[29] Shulman Lp, Muram D. Lack of heritability in ovarian germ cell malignancies. Am J Obstet Gynecol. 1994; 170:1803-8.

[30] Heslan I, Leveque J, Horyn G et al. Immature teratoma of the ovary A propos de 3 observations Revue de la litterature et mise au point. J Gynecol Obstet Biol Reprod. 1994; 23:790-6.

[31] Moniaga NC, Randall LM. Malignant mixed ovarian germ cell tumor with embryonal component. Journal of Pediatric and Adolescent Gynecology. 2011;24 (1): 1-3.

[32] Gershenson DM. Management of ovarian germ cell tumors. J Clin Oncol. 2007;25:2538-2543.

[33] Calongos G, Ogino M, Kinuta T, Hori M, Mori T. Sister Mary Joseph Nodule as a First Manifestation of a Metastatic Ovarian Cancer. Case Reports in Obstetrics and Gynecology. 2016: 1087513.

[34] About I. Tumeurs germinales malignes de l'ovaire analyse commentee d'une serie de 26 cas vus au centre Claudius Regaud entre 1974 et 1989. These Med Toulouse III. 1992.

[35] Pectasides D, Pectasides E, Kassanos D. Germ cell tumors of the ovary. Cancer Treat Rev. 2008; 34: 427-41.

[36] Caubel P, Giovan Grandi V, Lasry S. Seminoma and pregnancy A new case report. J Gynecol Obstet Biol Reprod. 1989; 18:487-91.

[37] Bakri Y N, Ezzat A, Akhtar, Dohami, Zahrani. Malignant germ cell tumors of the ovary. Pregnancy considerations. Eur J Obstet Gynecol Reprod Biol. 2000;1:87-91.

[38] Kurman RJ, Norris HJ. Endodermal sinus tumor of the ovary: a clinical and pathologic analysis of 71 cases. Cancer 1976 ;38(6):2404-19.

[39] Emoto M, Obama H, Horiuchi S, Miyakawa T, Kawarabayashi T. Transvaginal color Doppler ultrasonic characterization of benign and malignant ovarian cystic teratomas and comparison with serum squamous cell carcinoma antigen. Cancer. 2000;10: 2298-304.

[40] Bazot M, Darai E, Nassar-Slaba J, Lafont C, Thomassin-Naggara I. Value of magnetic resonance imaging for the diagnosis of ovarian tumors: a review. J Comput Assist Tomogr. 2008; 32:712-23.

[41] Akram M, Shaaban AM, Rezvani M, Elsayes KM, Baskin H Jr, Mourad A et al. Ovarian Malignant Germ Cell Tumors: Cellular Classification and Clinical and Imaging Features. Radiographics. 2014 ;34(3):777-801.

[42] Gilles P. Malignant germinal tumours of the ovary: Analysis of surgical and medical practices. A propos de 62 cas traites au centre Leon Berard et a l'institut Curie. Th D Med; Montpellier I; 2004.

[43] Fabiola M, Kyle CS. Germ Cell Tumors of the Ovary. Diagnostic Gynecologic and Obstetric Pathology. 2018; 949-1010.

[44] Parkinson CA, Hatcher HM, Ajithkumar TV. Management of malignant ovarian germ cell tumors. Obstet Gynecol Surv. 2011;66:507-514.

[45] NCCN Clinical Practice Guidelines in Oncology: Ovarian Cancer 2013.

[46] Talerman A. Germ cell tumors of the ovary. Blaustein's pathology of the female genital tract. 5th ed. New York, NY: Springer, 2002; 1391.

[47] Mahdi H, Kumar S, Seward S, et al. Prognostic impact of laterality in malignant ovarian germ cell tumors. Int J Gynecol Cancer. 2011;21(2):257-262.

[48] Capito C, Arnaud A, Hameury F, et al. Dysgerminoma and gonadal dysgenesis: the need for a new diagnosis tree for suspected ovarian tumours. J Pediatr Urol. 2011;7(3):367-372.

[49] Kurman RJ, Norris HJ. Embryonal carcinoma of the ovary: a clinicopathologic entity distinct from endodermal sinus tumor resembling embryonal carcinoma of the

adult testis. Cancer. 1976;38(6): 2420-2433.
[50] Ulbright TM. Germ cell tumors of the gonads: a selective review emphasizing problems in differential diagnosis, newly appreciated, and controversial issues. Mod Pathol. 2005;18(Suppl 2):S61-S79.
[51] Cheng L, Zhang S, Talerman A, Roth LM. Morphologic, immunohistochemical, and fluorescence in situ hybridization study of ovarian embryonal carcinoma with comparison to solid variant of yolk sac tumor and immature teratoma. Hum Pathol. 2010; 41(5):716-723.
[52] Jondle DM, Shahin MS, Sorosky J, Benda JA. Ovarian mixed germ cell tumor with predominance of polyembryoma: a case report with literature review. Int J Gynecol Pathol. 2002;21(1):78-81.
[53] Baker PM, Oliva E. Germ cell tumors of the ovary. Gynecologic pathology. 2009;501-538.
[54] Yanai-Inbar I, Scully RE. Relation of ovarian dermoid cysts and immature teratomas: an analysis of 350 cases of immature teratoma and 10 cases of dermoid cyst with microscopic foci of immature tissue. Int J Gynecol Pathol. 1987;6(3): 203-212.
[55] Noun M, Ennachit m, Boufettal h, Elmouatacim k, Samouh N. The ovarian immature teratoma with gliomatosis peritonei. Journal de Gynecologie Obstetrique et Biologie de la Reproduction. 2007; 36:595-601.
[56] Woodward PJ, Hosseinzadeh K, Saenger JS. From the archives of the AFIP: radiologic staging of ovarian carcinoma with pathologic correlation. RadioGraphics. 2004;24(1):225-246.
[57] Chen V, Ruiz B, Killeen JL, Cote T, Wu X, Correa C. Pathology and classification of ovarian tumors. Cancer. 2003;97(10):2631-2642.
[58] Jonathan B, Sean K, Lalit K, Michael F. Cancer of the ovary, fallopian tube, and peritoneum. FIGO cancer report 2018. 2018;143(2):59-78.
[59] Wollner N, Exelby Dr, Woodruff Jm et al. Malignant ovarian tumors in childhood. Cancer. 1976; 37: 1953-64.
[60] Pizzo Pa, Poplock DG. Principles and practice of pediatric oncology. 4th ed. Philadelphia; Lippincott Williams & Wlikins 2002: 6; 1-12.
[61] Billmire B. Outcome and staging evaluation in malignant germ cell tumors of the ovary in children and adolescents: an intergroup study. J Pediatr Surg. 2004; 3:424-9.
[62] Weinstein D. The role of wedge resection of the ovary as a cause of mechanical sterility. Surg Gynecol Obstet. 1975;141:417-8.
[64] Buttram Vc. Post ovarian wedge resection adhesive disease. Fertil Steril. 1975; 26:874-6.
[65] Monica T, Maura M, Michela C. Childhood Malignant Ovarian Germ Cell Tumors: A Monoinstitutional Experience. Gynecol Oncol 2001; 81: 436-40.
[66] Sagae S, Sasaki H, Nishioka Y, Terasawa K, Kudo R. Reproductive function after treatment of malignant germ cell ovarian tumors. Mol Cell Endocrinol. 2003; 202:117-21.

[67] El Lamie Ik, Shehata Na, Abou-Loz Sk, El-Lamie Ki. Conservative surgical management of malignant ovarian germ cell tumors: the experience of the Gynecologic Oncology Unit at Ain Shams University. Eur J Gynaecol Oncol. 2000; 6:605-9.

[68] Terenziani M, Massimino M, Casanova M et al. Childhood malignant ovarian germ cell tumors: a monoinstitutional experience. Gynecol Oncol. 2001; 81:436-40.

[69] Gadducci A, Cosio S, Muraca S, Genazzani A. The management of malignant nondysgerminomatous ovarian germ cell tumors. Anticancer Res 2003; 23:1827-36.

[70] Tangir J. Reproductive function after conservative surgery and chemotherapy for malignant germ cell tumors of the ovary. Obstet Gynecol. 2003; 101:251-7.

[71] Lin KY, Bryant S, Miller DS, Kehoe SM, Richardson DL, Lea JS. Malignant ovarian germ cell tumor-role of surgical staging and gonadal dysgenesis. Gynecol Oncol. 2014;134:84-9.

[72] Ibrahim E, Salih T, Rifat G, Muzaffer B, Goksu G, Yusuf Y et al. Longterm oncological and reproductive outcomes of fertility-sparing cytoreductive surgery in females aged 25 years and younger with malignant ovarian germ cell tumors. J Obstet Gynaecol Res. 2014;40(3):797-805.

[73] Lu KH, Gershenson DM. Update on the management of ovarian germ cell tumors. J Reprod Med. 2005;50:417-25.

[74] Ki Heon L, In Ho L, Byoung Gie K, Joo Hyun N, Won Kyu K, Soon Beom K et al. Clinicopathologic characteristics of malignant germ cell tumors in the ovaries of Korean women: a Korean Gynecologic Oncology Group Study. Int J Gynecol Cancer. 2009;19:84-7.

[75] Siriwan T, Jitti H, Sumonmal M et al. Malignant ovarian germ cell tumors: clinico-pathological presentation and survival outcomes. Acta Obstet Gynecol Scand. 2010;89(2):182-9.

[76] Palenzuela G, Martin E, Meunier A, Beuzeboc P, Laurence V, Daniel O et al. Comprehensive staging allows for excellent outcome in patients with localized malignant germ cell tumor of the ovary. Ann Surg. 2008;248:836-41.

[77] Kleppe M, Amkreutz LC, Van Gorp T et al. Lymph-node metastasis in stage I and II sex cord stromal and malignant germ cell tumours of the ovary: a systematic review. Gynecol Oncol. 2014;133:124-7.

[78] Geisler J, Goulet R, Foster R, Sutton G. Growing teratoma syndrome after chemotherapy for germ cell tumors of the ovary. Obstet Gynecol. 1994; 84: 71921.

[79] Andre F, Fizazi K, Culine S. The growing teratoma syndrome: results of therapy and longterm fol-low-up of 33 patients. Eur J Cancer. 2000; 36: 138994.

[80] Williams S, Blessing J, Moore D, Homesley H, Adcock L. Cisplatin, vinblastine and bleomycin in advanced and recurrent ovarian germ cell tumors. Ann Intern Med. 1989;111:22-7.

[81] Slayton RE, Park RC, Silverberg SG, Shingleton H, Creasman WT, Blessing JA. Vincristine, dactinomycin and cyclophosphamide in the treatment of malignant germ cell tumors of the ovary. A Gynecologic Oncology Group Study (a final report).

Cancer. 1985;56:243-8.
[82] Jin Li, PhD, Xiaohua Wu. Current Strategy for the Treatment of Ovarian Germ Cell Tumors: Role of Extensive Surgery. Curr. Treat. Options in Oncol. 2016; 17:44.
[83] Gershenson DM, Del Junco G, Herson J, Rutledge F. Endodermal sinus tumor of the ovary: the M. D. Anderson experience. Obstet Gynecol. 1983;61 (2):194-202.
[84] Gallion H, VanNagell R, Powell F, Donaldson D, Hanson M. Therapy of endodermal sinus tumor of the ovary. Am J Obstet Gynecol. 1979;135: 447451.
[85] Gershenson D, Copeland L, Kavanagh J, Cangir A et al. Treatment of malignant non dysgerminomatous germ cell tumors of the ovary with vincristine, dactinomycin, and cyclophosphamide. Cancer. 1985;56 (12): 27562761.
[86] Einhorn LH, Donohue J. Cis-diamminedi-chloroplatinum, vinblastine, and bleomycin combination chemotherapy in disseminated testicular cancer. Ann Intern Med. 1977;87:293-298.
[87] Julian CB, Barrett J, Richardson R, Greco F. Bleomycin, vinblastine, and cisplatinum in the treatment of advanced endodermal sinus tumor. Obstet Gynecol. 1980;56: 396-401.
[88] Williams SD, Birch R, Einhorn L, Irwin L, Greco F, Loehrer P. Treatment of disseminated germ-cell tumors with cisplatin, bleomycin, and either vinblastine or etoposide. N Engl J Med. 1987;316 (23) :1435-1440.
[89] Gershenson D, Morris M, Cangir A, Kavanagh A, Stringer C et al. Treatment of malignant germ cell tumors of the ovary with bleomycin, etoposide, and cisplatin. J Clin Oncol. 1990;8 (4):715-720.
[90] Brewer M, Gershenson DM, Herzog CE, Mitchell MF, Silva E, Wharton J. Outcome and reproductive function after chemotherapy for ovarian dysgerminoma. J Clin Oncol. 1999;17 (9): 2670-2675.
[91] Gershenson DM. Current advances in the management of malignant germ cell and sex cord-stromal tumors of the ovary. Gynecol Oncol 2012;125(3): 515-517.
[92] Colombo N, Peiretti M, Castiglione M. Non-epithelial ovarian cancer: ESMO clinical recommendations for diagnosis, treatment and follow-up. Ann Oncol. 2009;20:24-26.
[93] Cushing B, Giller R, Cullen J, Marina N, Lauer S, Olson TA et al. Randomized comparison of combination chemotherapy with etoposide, bleomycin, and either high dose or standard dose cisplatin in children and adolescents with high risk malignant germ cell tumors: a pediatric intergroup study- Pediatric Oncology Group 9049 and Children's Cancer Group 8882. J Clin Oncol. 2004; 39: 2691-700.
[94] Einhorn LH, Williams SD, Chamness A et al. High-dose chemotherapy and stem-cell rescue for metastatic germ-cell tumors. N Engl J Med. 2007;357:340- 348.
[95] Ovarian Germ Cell Tumors (PDF). April 2013. Retrieved 2019-04-01.
[96] Manchana T, Ittiwut C, Mutirangura A. Targeted therapies for rare gynaecological cancers. Lancet Oncol 2010; 117: 685-693.
[97] Lai CH, Chang TC, Hsueh S, Wu TI, Chao A, Chou HH. Outcome and prognostic factors in ovarian germ cell malignancies. Gynecol Oncol. 2005;

96(3):784-91.
[98] Germ Cell and Nonepithelial Ovarian Cancer. Oncohema Key. 2016.
[99] Jeyakumar A, Cabeza R, Hindenburg A. Late recurrence in ovarian dysgerminoma with successful response to standard adjuvant chemotherapy: a case report and review of the literature. Gynecol Oncol. 2001; 81:314-7.
[100] Dubrex. Histopathologie Gynecologique. 2eme ed. Paris: Masson 1982; 12: 378-406.
[101] Masmoudi M. Etude anatomo-clinique des tumeurs germinales de l'ovaire. Th D Med ; Tunis ; 1993.
[102] Norris H, Zirkin Hj, Benson Wl. Immature malignant teratoma of the ovary A clinical and pathologic study of 58 cases. Cancer. 1976; 37:2359-72.
[103] Harada M, Osuga Y, Fujimoto A, Fujimoto A, Fujii T, Yano T, Kozuma S. Predictive factors for recurrence of ovarian mature cystic teratomas after surgical excision. Eur J Obstet Gynecol Reprod Biol. 2013; 171: 325-328.
[104] Jubilee B, MD, Michael F. Gynecologic Cancer Intergroup (GCIG) Consensus Review for Ovarian Germ Cell Tumors. Int J Gynecol Cancer. 2014;24: 48-54.
[105] Gershenson DM, Miller AM, Champion VL, et al. Reproductive and sexual function after platinum-based chemotherapy in long-term ovarian germ cell tumor survivors: a Gynecologic Oncology Group Study. J Clin Oncol. 2007;25:2792-2797.
[106] De La Motte Rouge T, Pautier P, Rey A, Duvillard P, Kerbrat P, Troalen F et al. Prognostic factors in women treated for ovarian yolk sac tumour: a retrospective analysis of 84 cases. Eur J Cancer Jan. 2011; 47:175-82.
[107] Zanagnolo V, Sartori E, Galleri G, Pasinetti B, Bianchi U. Clinical review of 55 cases of malignant ovarian germ cell tumors. Eur J Gynaecol Oncol. 2004; 3:315-20.
[108] Low J, Perrin LC, Crandon AJ et al. Conservative surgery to preserve ovarian function in patients with malignant ovarian germ cell tumors. A review of 74 cases. Cancer. 2000; 89: 391-398.
[109] Zanetta G, Bonazzi C, Cantu M et al. Survival and reproductive function after treatment of malignant germ cell ovarian tumors. J Clin Oncol. 2001;19:1015-1020.
[110] Rousset-Jablonski C, Selle F, Adda-Herzog E, Planchamp F, Selleret L, Pomel C et al. Fertility preservation, contraception and hormonal treatment of menopause in women treated for rare malignant ovarian tumours: recommendations of the national network dedicated to rare gynecological cancers (TMRG/GINECO). Bull Cancer. 2018; 105: 299-314.
[111] Survival rates for ovarian cancer, by stage. American Cancer Society. Archived from the original on 29 October 2014. Retrieved 29 October 2014.
[112] Gershenson DM. Current advances in the management of malignant germ cell and sex cord-stromal tumors of the ovary. Gynecol Oncol. 2012;125(3): 515-517.
[113] Jorge S, Jones N, Chen L, Hou JY, Tergas AI, Burke W et al. Characteristics, treatment and outcomes of women with immature ovarian Teratoma, 1998-2012. Gynecologic oncology. 2016; 142: 261-6.
[114] Baranzelli MC, Kramar A, Bouffet E, Quintana E, Rubie H, Edan C et al.

Prognostic Factors in Children With Localized Malignant Nonseminomatous Germ Cell Tumors. J Clin Oncol. 1999;17:1212-8.
[115] Nawa A, Obata N, Kikkawa F, Kawai M, Nagasaka T, Goto S et al. Prognostic factors of patients with yolk sac tumors of the ovary. Am J Obstet Gynecol. 2001; 184 : 1182-8.
[116] Cicin I, Saip P, Guney N, Eralp Y, Ayan I, Kebudi R et al. Yolk sac tumours of the ovary: evaluation of clinicopathological features and prognostic factors. Eur J Obstet Gynecol Reprod Biol. 2009; 146 : 210-4.
[117] Stephen D, James K, Alexander F, Samuel S, Karol A, Deborah K. Adjuvant therapy of completely resected dysgerminoma with carboplatin and etoposide: a trial of the Gynecologic Oncology Group. Gynecol Oncol. 2004; 95: 496-9.
[118] Jin F, Zhu G, Feng YJ. Clinical features and prognostic factors of malignant ovarian teratoma. Zhongguo Yi Xue Ke Xue Yuan Xue Bao 2003; 25:427-30.
[119] Kildal W, Kaern J, Kraggerud S, Abeler V, Sudbo J, Trope C et al. Evaluation of genomic changes in a large series of malignant ovarian germ cell tumors--relation to clinicopathologic variables. Cancer Genet Cytogenet. 2004; 155:25-32.
[120] Tewari K, Cappuccini F, Disaia PJ, Berman ML, Manetta A, Kohler MF. Malignant germ cell tumors of the ovary. Obstet Gynecol. 2000; 95: 128-33.
[121] Slayton RE. Management of germ cell and stromal tumors of the ovary. Semin Oncol. 1984;11:299-313.
[122] Kumar S, Shah J, Bryant C, Imudia A, Cote M, Ali-Fehmi R et al. The prevalence and prognostic impact of lymph node metastasis in malignant germ cell tumours of the ovary. Gynecol Oncol. 2008;110:125-32.
[123] Madhi H, Swensen RE, Hanna E, Kumar S, Ali-Fehmi R, Semaan A et al. Prognostic impact of lymphadenectomy in clinical early stage malignant germ cell tumour of the ovary. Br J Cancer. 2011;105:493-7.
[124] Liu Q, Ding X, Yang J, Cao D, Shen K, Lang J, et al. The significance of comprehensive staging surgery in malignant ovarian germ cell tumors. Gynecol Oncol. 2013;131:551-4.
[125] Chan JK, Tewari KS, Waller S. The influence of conservative surgical practices for malignant ovarian germ cell tumors. J Surg Oncol. 2008; 98:111-6.
[126] Aizer AA, Chen MH, McCarthy EP, et al. Marital status and survival in patients with cancer. J Clin Oncol. 2013; 31:3869-3876.
[127] Solheim O, Kaern J, Trope C, Rokkones E, Dahl A, Nesland J et al. Malignant ovarian germ cell tumors: presentation, survival and second cancer in a population based Norwegian cohort (1953-2009). Gynecol Oncol. 2013;131: 330-335.
[128] Leblanc P, Coche-Dequant B, Querleu D, Raviart S, Grepin G. Le dysgerminome ovarien Actualite diagnostique et therapeutique. Rev Fr Gynecol Obstet. 1988 ; 83 :51-61.

7 APPENDIX

Annex I

DATA SHEET

SHEET NO. :

A- IDENTIFICATION AND ANTECEDENTS

Last name : First name :

Date of birth :

Origin : 1 Sousse 2 Non Sousse

Marital status: 1 Single 2 Married 3 Divorced 4 No, please specify :

Age of the first regies :

Gestite :

Parite :

Menopause: 1 No, 2 Yes_ If Yes age at menopause :

Contraception: 1 No 2 Yes_ If Yes type of contraception 1: Hormonal, 2 Non Hormonal

Medical history: 0: No, 1: Yes_ If yes, please specify:

Previous surgery: 0: No, 1: Yes_ If Yes, please specify:

Family history of cancer: 0: No, 1: Yes_ If yes, please specify:

Personal history of cancer : 0 : No 1: Yes_ If yes, please specify :

B- CLINICAL SYMPTOMS

Consultation deadline :

Date of 1st symptom :

Date of 1st consultation :

Circumstances of discovery :

1 : Metrorragies
2 Dysmenorrhea
3 Infertility
4 Abdominal and/or pelvic pain
5 : Increase in abdominal volume
6 : Change in general condition
7 Pelvic and/or abdominal mass
8 Urinary disorders
9 Transit disorders
10 Accidental discovery: 0 No, 1 Yes_ If Yes, please specify:

C- BIOLOGY

- High rate of CA125 : 0 : No 1: Yes, If Yes specify value :
- High rate of AFP : 0: No 1 : Yes, If Yes specify value :
- High HCG level: 0: No, 1: Yes, If Yes specify value:
- High LDH level: 0: No, 1: Yes, If Yes specify value:

D- PELVIC ULTRASOUND

Location : 1: Right ovary, 2: Left ovary, 3: Bilateral

*RIGHT OVARY :

1 pure anechoic image, 2 echogenic image, 3 heterogeneous image

4 partition , 5 vegetation , 6 clean wall , 7 doppler plug , 8 size in mm

*LEFT OVARY :

1 pure anechoic image , 2 echoic image , 3 heterogeneous image

4 partition , 5 vegetation , 6 clean wall , 7 doppler plug , 8 size in mm

*UTERUS :

height (mm) :

width (mm) :
*ENDOMETER :
thickness (mm) : , echogene , hypoechoene , hyper echogene
*LATCH IN DOUGLAS: 0: No, 1: Yes, If Yes specify size in mm
* NODULES IN DOUGLAS : 0: No, 1 : Yes , If Yes specify size in mm

E- THORACO-ABDOMINO-PELVIC TDM

*RIGHT OVARY :
hypodense image, hyperdense image, heterogeneous image , contrast yes or no partition , vegetation , clean wall , size in mm :
* LEFT OVARY :
hypodense image, hyperdense image, heterogeneous image, contrast enhancement yes or no partition, vegetation , clean wall , size in mm
* UTERUS :
height in mm :
width in mm :
* ENDOMETER :
thickness (mm) , density
* EPANCHEMENT: 0: no , 1: yes , if yes specify if it is enclosed or free , and abundance of effusion
*PERITONEAL NODULE: 0: no , 1: yes , if yes specify size in mm
*DIGESTIVE NODULES: 0: no , 1: yes , if yes specify size in mm
*VESICAL NODULES: 0: no , 1: yes , if yes specify size in mm
*ASPECTS OF THE URETERS :
*MESENTERIC GRANLIONS: 0: no , 1: yes , if yes specify number , right or left , pelvic or lumbo-aortic
* HEPATIC NODULES: 0: no , 1: yes , if yes specify number
* PULMONARY NODULES: 0: no , 1: yes , if yes specify number
* THORACIC ADP: 0: no , 1: yes , if yes specify number
* FLOORING: 0: no , 1: yes , if yes specify, right, left or bilateral and abundance

F- PELVIC MRI

*RIGHT OVARY :
hyposignal , hypersignal , heterogeneous image , septum , vegetation , clean wall , size in mm :
*LEFT OVARY :
hyposignal , hypersignal , heterogeneous image , septum , vegetation , clean wall , size in mm
* UTERUS :
height in mm :
width in mm :
* ENDOMETER :
thickness (mm) , density
* EPANCHEMENT: 0: no , 1: yes , if yes specify if it is enclosed or free , and abundance of effusion
*PERITONEAL NODULE: 0: no , 1: yes , if yes specify size in mm
*DIGESTIVE NODULES: 0: no , 1: yes , if yes specify size in mm
*VESICAL NODULES: 0: no , 1: yes , if yes specify size in mm
*ASPECTS OF THE URETERS :
*MESENTERIC GRANLIONS: 0: no , 1: yes , if yes specify number , right or left , pelvic or lumbo-aortic
* HEPATIC NODULES: 0: no , 1: yes , if yes specify number
* PULMONARY NODULES: 0: no , 1: yes , if yes specify number

* THORACIC ADP: 0: no , 1: yes , if yes specify number
* FLOORING: 0: no , 1: yes , if yes specify, right, left or bilateral and abundance

G- ASCITES PUNCTURE

0: No, 1 : Yes_ If Yes cytology result :

H-C(DIAGNOSTIC ELIOSCOPY

Date of crelioscopy in relation to 1st consultation:

*RIGHT OVARY :

solid mass , cystic , solidokystic

partition , vegetation , clean wall , size in mm

*LEFT OVARY :

solid mass , cystic , solidokystic

partition , vegetation , clean wall , size in mm

* UTERUS :

height in mm

width in mm

* LEAKAGE: 0: no ,1: yes ,if yes partitioned or free, amount of leakage
* PERITONEAL NODULE: 0: no , 1: yes , if yes specify location and size in mm
* DIGESTIVE NODULES: 0: no , 1: yes ,if yes specify location and size in mm
* VESICAL NODULES: 0: no , 1: yes , if yes specify location and size in mm
* HEPATIC NODULES: 0: no , 1: yes ,if yes specify location and size in mm

STADIFICATION : 1: Ia , 2: Ib , 3: Ic , 4: IIa , 5: IIb , 6: IIc , 7 : IIIa , 8: IIIb , 9 IIIc , 10 IV

GESTURES :

*Peritoneal cytology: 0: no , 1: yes

* Right ovary biopsy: 0: no , 1: yes
* Left ovarian biopsy: 0: no , 1: yes
* Right cystectomy: 0: no , 1: yes
* Left cystectomy: 0: no , 1: yes
* Right adnexectomy 0: no , 1 : yes
* Left adnexectomy 0: no , 1 : yes
* Hysterectomy : 0: no , 1 : yes
* Omentectomy: 0: no , 1: yes
* Appendiectomy : 0: no , 1 : yes
* Parietal nodule resection or parietal nodule biopsy: 0: no , 1: yes
* Action on the digestive tract: 0: no , 1: yes
* Gesture on the ureters: 0: no , 1: yes
* Lymph node dissection: 0: no , 1: yes if yes pelvic only , lomboaortic only or pelvic and lomboaortic

I- ANATOMY AND PATHOLOGY

Date of histological diagnosis :

*MACROSCOPY :

-Location : 1: Right ovary , 2 : Left ovary , 3 Bilateral

- Size in mm :
- Consistency : 1 Solid , 2 : Cystic , 3 : Solid-cystic
- vegetation or partition :
- Stage : 1: pIa , 2: pIb , 3: pIc , 4: pIIa , 5: pIIb , 6: pIIc , 7 : pIIIa , 8: pIIIb , 9 pIIIc , 10 pIV

*MICROSCOPY :

- Histological type :
- Histological grade : 1: Grade I , 2: Grade II , 3 : Grade III
- Degree of differentiation :

- Immunohistochemistry :

J- TREATMENT

Date of surgery :
Duration of the act :
Type of anaesthesia :
SURGERY : 0: No 1: Yes, If Yes please specify

- surgical approach : 1 : coelio , 2 : laparo , 3 :laparo conversion
- surgical procedure : 1 : single or bilateral ovary , 2 : ovary + uterus , 3 : ovary + uterus + epiplon , 4 : ovary + uterus + epiplon + appdecicetomy
- gum removal :

-curage route: 1: coelio or 2: laparo
-type of curage: 1: pelvic 1 uni or 2 bilateral, 2: lomboaortic 1 uni or 2 bilateral, 3: pelvic and lomboaortic 1 uni or 2 bilateral.
*duration of hospitalisation for surgery :

* post-surgery tumour residue: 0: no , 1: yes , if yes size in mm and location
* Drain de Redon : 0: no , 1 : yes , si oui uni ou bilateral
* Date ablation redon :
* Surgical complications: 0: no , 1: yes , if yes specify :

1: infection, 2: delayed healing, 3: thromboembolic accident, 4: urinary infection, 5: bladder wound, 6: digestive wound

* Transufusion: 0: no, 1: yes, if yes per or post op, number of packed red blood cells
* Complications of anaesthesia :

CHEMOTHERAPY :

* Neoadjuvant: 0: no, 1: yes
* Adjuvant: 0: no, 1: yes

*Protocol :
*Number of treatments :

* Start date :
* End date :
* Chemotherapy complications: nausea vomiting aplasia neutropenia anemia
* Post chemotherapy imaging:

post-chemotherapy response ,
tumour residue, if so specify in mm

* Post chemo biology: Tumour markers :
* post-chemotherapy response :

tumour residue yes no , if yes in mm
2 LOOK SURGERY: 0: no , 1: yes, if yes postivie or negative
post-tumour residue: 0: no , 1: yes, if yes size and location

K-EVOLUTION AND MONITORING

- METASTASE: 0: no, 1: yes_ if yes, specify location and date of discovery and reason for discovery

1: hepatic, 2: pleural , 3 gonglion de troisier , 4 : Diaphragmatic

- RECIDENCE: 0: no , 1: yes , if yes specify date size and circumstances of discovery
- FERTILITY : 0: infertile, spontaneous fertility, fertility under MAP
- CURRENT STATUS: 1: living in remission , 2: living in progress , 3: lost from sight , 4 : deceased if yes date of death
- CAUSE OF DEATH: 1: progression, 2: other :

Title: II MALIGNANT GERMINAL TUMEURS OF THE OVAIRE: ASPECTS CLINICO-PATHOLOGICAL, THERAPEUTIC AND PROGNOSTIC FACTORS.

SUMMARY

Introduction: Germ cell tumours of the ovary are the most common rare ovarian tumours and are estimated to account for 6% of all ovarian tumours. They arise from primordial germ cells and are composed of several tumour types. Each histological type may have specific clinical, biological, anatomopathological and/or therapeutic features that it is important to be aware of. The degree of malignancy differs between the different histological types. The reported 5-year survival rates also differ.

Materials and methods: Our study is a retrospective descriptive and analytical study carried out in the Gynecology-Obstetrics, Medical Oncology and Anatomopathology Departments of the FARHAT HACHED University Hospital in Sousse over a period of 21 years (1st September 1998 to 30th September 2019), collating all cases of patients treated for malignant germ cell tumours of the ovary.

Objectives: -To report and analyse the epidemiological, diagnostic, anatomopathological, therapeutic and prognostic features of malignant germ cell tumours of the ovary. - To compare our results with those of the literature and to propose a decisional diagram which could improve the management of this entity in our Tunisian context.

Results: A total of 30 cases were eligible for our study. The mean age of our patients was 22 years, with extremes ranging from 10 to 40 years. The majority of patients (93.3%) were genitally active, two-thirds of whom were nulliparous. The average consultation time was less than 6 months in 70% of cases. The main reason for consultation was abdomino-pelvic pain in 45% of cases, followed by an increase in abdominal volume in 17% of cases. Abdominopelvic ultrasound was performed in 80% of our patients, showing a suspicious appearance of malignancy in 100%. The most characteristic appearance was a heterogeneous parenchymal echogenic mass with sharp margins and high vascularity.

For our patients, 70% were approached by median laparotomy, given the volume of the tumour, and only 30% by calioscopy. 76.7% underwent conservative treatment. Lymph node surgery was performed in only 10% of our patients. Stage I was predominant in 17 patients (56.7%), stage II in 2 (6.7%), stage III in 11 (36.7%), and stage IV in none. Complementary treatment to surgery in the form of poly-chemotherapy was indicated in 24 patients (80%). The BEP protocol was used in 85.7% of cases.

We observed continued progression in one patient and 3 cases of metastatic recurrence. Salvage treatment consisted of second-line chemotherapy in all cases. Mean survival in the study population was 94 months. Overall survival for all stages was 96.7% at 2 years, 85.7% at 5 years and 75.8% at 10 years. Overall survival at 20 years was 56.4%.

The prognostic factors for the isolated malignant germ cell tumours of the ovary in our series were a consultation time of more than 6 months, age of more than 30 years, tumour size of more than 20 cm and tumour stage. Among 10 women attempting pregnancy, 9 were able to conceive, 2 of whom were stage III at the time of diagnosis, thus confirming that conservative treatment should be recommended even at advanced stages.

CONCLUSION: Although the size of this study is small, the results appear to be consistent with larger series. However, it would be more interesting to collect the other cases of TGMO diagnosed at the level of the other cancer registries in the country in order to establish a national series of this tumour, within the framework of a national registry of rare ovarian tumours.

Key words : II *Ovary, Malignant germ cell tumours, Radical surgery, Surgery Conservative* II, *Chemotherapy, Survival, Fertility.*

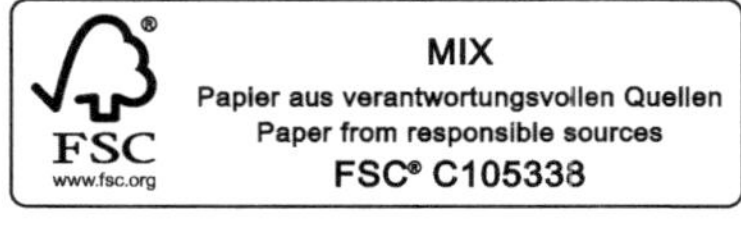

Printed by Books on Demand GmbH, Norderstedt / Germany